Strong as a Mother

STRONG AS A

FOUNDERS OF 4TWO
Shannon Rowbury &
Jessica Dorrington
MPT, OCS, PRPC

YOUR COMPLETE
PREGNANCY-TO-
POSTPARTUM
HEALTH PROGRAM

MOTHER

SASQUATCH BOOKS | SEATTLE

For all the strong moms and their strong girls

Contents

Your Journey to Strength

YOU ARE STRONG AS A MOTHER

Welcome to your journey of strength and discovery through pregnancy and beyond. This book is designed to be your companion and to support your needs as you navigate this transformative period.

The Four-Trimester Approach

Our journey together spans the traditional three trimesters of pregnancy plus the crucial "fourth trimester"—the first three months of your postpartum period. This comprehensive approach ensures that you're supported from conception through your recovery and return to movement, whatever that looks like for you.

Every pregnancy journey is unique, as is every person's relationship with physical activity. Our exercise program is designed to meet you where you are, supporting your changing body through each stage of pregnancy. Think of each trimester as a distinct phase of your journey, each with its own goals and opportunities for growth.

FIRST TRIMESTER: BUILDING YOUR FOUNDATION

During these early weeks, we focus on establishing good movement patterns and breathing techniques to help you build the foundational strength you'll need throughout your pregnancy. Energy levels often fluctuate, so we've designed these initial exercises to be manageable yet effective whether you're continuing an existing fitness routine or starting fresh.

SECOND TRIMESTER: GROWING STRONGER

Many women find renewed energy during this phase. Whether you're experienced with exercise or new to regular movement, we'll help you make the most of this typically energetic phase while maintaining safety. You'll build on your established foundation and progress to more dynamic movements as you adapt to your changing center of gravity.

THIRD TRIMESTER: PREPARING FOR BIRTH

As your belly grows, your movement patterns change, and birth preparation becomes essential. We'll help you modify your movements to maintain strength and stability. In Chapter 13's birth preference plan, you'll find advice on birthing positions, partner roles, birth center prep, and much more.

FOURTH TRIMESTER: RECOVERING AND PROSPERING

This postpartum period requires a thoughtful approach to movement and recovery. We'll guide you through the early postpartum days all the way back to your favorite activities with detailed exercise plans and return-to-fitness checklists, all while respecting your body's healing process.

Special Features Throughout the Book

WELLNESS FOCUS BOXES

Look for these highlighted sections to find key concepts, practical applications, complementary support, and quick reference points that you can easily return to throughout your pregnancy journey.

FROM THE PRO

Throughout the book, you'll find personal insights that bring our guidance to life. While Shannon shares stories from her Olympic career and her transition to motherhood, Jessica offers clinical expertise and observations from years of working with pregnant and postpartum clients. You'll also find testimonials from other Olympic athletes sharing their experiences navigating sport alongside pregnancy and postpartum life. These real-world perspectives provide practical strategies to help you overcome common challenges and adapt to your changing needs.

SAFETY FIRST

Your safety is our top priority, which is why each chapter contains comprehensive safety information. We outline what to watch for during exercise, including specific warning signs that indicate when to modify your activity or contact your healthcare provider. You'll find detailed guidelines to help you adapt your movements as needed, ensuring you can stay active while respecting your limits. We've designed these safety elements to help you exercise confidently and make informed decisions about your well-being.

Making the Most of Your Journey

TRACKING YOUR PROGRESS

We encourage you to keep a pregnancy journal as you move through this experience. Think of it as a conversation with yourself about your changing body and evolving needs. Take time to note how you're feeling each day, including your energy levels and how different movements affect you. Write down any questions that arise for your health-care providers—no detail is too small. By documenting both your physical achievements and emotional responses throughout this journey, you'll create an invaluable record to track your progress and reflect on your incredible strength and adaptability during pregnancy. Plus, your journal can be a great resource to refer to during future pregnancies.

EXERCISE PROGRAMS

Each trimester includes multiple variations of exercises, for all ability levels, timed intentionally to support your body throughout pregnancy. These exercises will also play an important role during your postpartum recovery, so getting familiar with them now will save you steps down the road.

We encourage you to approach your fitness journey with patience and mindfulness, even if you're already physically active. Start with the fundamentals and take your time to master proper form before progressing to more challenging movements. Each repetition reinforces movement patterns, so focusing on good form and technique early on will pay off in the later weeks.

Remember, your body will communicate with you differently each day during pregnancy—honor these signals and adjust your workout intensity as needed. Rest days are essential strategic pauses that allow your body to recover and grow stronger.

MEET YOUR GUIDES: SHANNON ROWBURY & JESSICA DORRINGTON

We wrote this book to give women confidence in how they approach physical health during pregnancy and postpartum. One of the first questions many pregnant women have is, "How can I stay healthy and active while nurturing this new life inside me?" Coming from different professional backgrounds, we each approached this question from a unique angle. Despite this, we arrived at the same conclusion: Pregnant bodies are capable of more than traditional advice suggests.

Shannon Rowbury: Bridging Olympic Excellence and Motherhood

For over a decade, I've pushed the boundaries of what's possible on the track. As a three-time Olympian, Olympic medalist, and world record holder, I've experienced the pinnacle of athletic achievement. However, it wasn't until I became pregnant with my daughter Sienna in 2017 that I faced my most challenging and rewarding "event" yet.

When I first learned that I was pregnant, I was terrified. Over a decade as a professional athlete, I'd witnessed other athlete moms lose their health insurance, deal with contract reductions, and end their athletic careers due to the lack of financial support. The professional running world hadn't made space for athlete moms who wanted to continue competing after growing their families. Fortunately, my coach, Pete Julian, and my strength coach, Dave McHenry, were incredibly supportive throughout my pregnancy journey. I waited until twenty weeks to share the news publicly, but Pete and Dave were among the first to know, and through them I met Jessica Dorrington.

With Jessica's help, I chose a balanced approach to staying active during pregnancy. After a decade of intense training, I understood the toll it had taken on my body and didn't want to add to that while growing a baby. My primary goal became a healthy pregnancy.

The hardest part was stepping back and letting my body's pregnancy autopilot take over. As a competitor, I was used to honing my body into peak fitness—workout after workout, week after week—developing such control that I could hit race pace within five steps of an interval. During pregnancy, however, my body's greatest accomplishment—creating a new life—required me to relinquish control. I'll never forget how Sienna would kick and punch whenever my pants were too tight; she kicked with such fervor that it eventually created a hole in my amniotic sac! All I could do was buy bigger pants.

After Sienna's birth, I faced some initial postpartum setbacks. But in the end I didn't just return to competition—I thrived. I qualified for the US Olympic Trials, ran the Olympic standard, and set the US Masters record for the 5K. My pregnancy journey taught me that motherhood and athletic excellence aren't mutually exclusive. They can, in fact, beautifully complement each other.

MENTAL AND EMOTIONAL SUPPORT:
Your mental and emotional wellness will receive equal attention through evidence-based stress management techniques, meaningful self-reflection activities, and mindfulness practices that create calm amid the excitement and uncertainty of pregnancy. You'll optimize sleep and prepare mentally for birth with confidence-building strategies that are rooted in athletic performance and maternal health expertise.

Community and Support

Having the right support during pregnancy and postpartum can make all the difference, starting with your healthcare team. We encourage you to share this book with your healthcare providers and use it as a tool to guide your conversations about staying active during pregnancy.

Beyond your medical team, building a support network can provide comfort and encouragement throughout your journey. Try connecting with other expecting parents through local groups or by joining our online community. Family and friends might also be able to offer emotional support and practical help. Thoughtfully choosing your birth team and finding healthcare providers who align with your preferences and goals can help you feel more confident and prepared. And as you move into the postpartum phase, having a plan

for support during those first weeks with your newborn will be invaluable, so plan ahead.

A PERSONAL JOURNEY

Pregnancy is a deeply personal experience. Listen to your body's wisdom as it guides you in making choices that feel right for you. Focus on celebrating each small victory along the way rather than striving for perfection. Our goal is to help you build a strong foundation that will serve you throughout your pregnancy, into motherhood, and beyond. You possess more strength than you might realize, and we hope this book can help you feel strong as a mother.

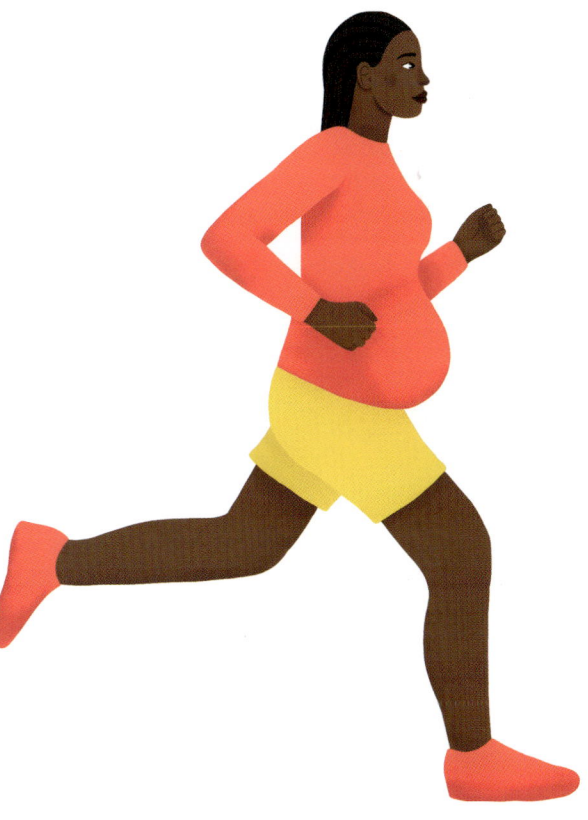

PART I

FOUNDATIONS OF PRENATAL FITNESS

CHAPTER 1

Why Traditional Pregnancy Advice Is Holding You Back

Not so long ago, the words "pregnancy" and "athletics" were rarely uttered in the same breath. If you were to rewind to just a few decades ago, you'd find a medical landscape where pregnant women were routinely advised to drastically limit physical activity. The prevailing wisdom prioritized caution above all else, even if it meant months of inactivity.

THE PROBLEM WITH PLAYING IT SAFE

Previous guidelines set by the American College of Obstetrics and Gynecology (ACOG) imposed strict parameters:

- Limitations on heart rate during exercise
- Restrictions on starting new activities for previously inactive mothers
- Prohibitions on movements deemed too risky

While these guidelines were well-intentioned, their overly cautious nature left many women feeling uncertain and even fearful about staying active during pregnancy. Fortunately, the medical community has begun to recognize the tremendous benefits of exercise during pregnancy for both parent and baby. ACOG reviews its physical activity guidelines for pregnancy annually and continues to update its protocols. The organization now recommends that pregnant women engage in at least 150 minutes of moderate-intensity aerobic activity per week—it's worth checking for updates each year. While pre-, peri-, and postpartum fitness remain relatively new fields in medicine, there have been noteworthy advancements in recent years.

THE CURRENT RESEARCH

Research shows that women who exercise during pregnancy experience remarkable benefits to their physical fitness. Compared to those who don't exercise, women who exercise during pregnancy:

- Retain three times less weight
- Retain two times less fat
- Experience significant improvement in abdominal tone
- Return to prepregnancy activity levels twice as often

But exercise during pregnancy isn't just about staying fit—it sets the stage for a healthier pregnancy, easier recovery, and a strong start to motherhood. Research consistently shows the health benefits that staying active during pregnancy provides for both mothers and their babies.

For mothers, exercise:
- Reduces the risk of gestational diabetes by 24 to 38 percent
- Enhances their ability to handle the physical demands of labor
- Lowers the likelihood of needing a cesarean delivery
- Improves psychological well-being and reduces the risk of depression during pregnancy and postpartum
- Promotes better postpartum recovery outcomes
- Eliminates or improves low back pain
- Improves muscular tone and posture

For babies, it:
- Improves placental growth, volume, and function
- Helps regulate the baby's weight
- Improves muscle tone
- Increases the likelihood of a vaginal delivery for beneficial bacterial exposure
- Promotes a potentially shorter labor
- Improves the baby's position for birth

Unfortunately, many women are still advised to limit or avoid exercise due to outdated information or fear. *It's time to challenge this narrative.*

BREAKING FREE FROM COMMON MYTHS

In this book, we'll challenge long-standing myths surrounding pregnancy, birth, and postpartum recovery. Some of these misconceptions have persisted for generations, affecting how women approach pregnancy and, in turn, what they think their bodies are capable of. Here's a glimpse at some of the beliefs we'll examine:

MYTH: You'll get all the guidance you need by listening to your body

Pregnancy changes everything, including the way your body communicates. But what does it really mean to listen to your body when pregnancy alters your usual feedback systems? We'll explore this complex relationship and provide clear guidance.

Jessica Dorrington: Combining Clinical Expertise with Real Experience

As a board-certified orthopedic and sports physical therapist specializing in pelvic health since 2002, I've had the privilege of guiding countless women through the physical transformations of pregnancy and postpartum recovery. My practice is about more than just treatment—it's about empowering women to embrace their changing bodies and maintain active, healthy lifestyles.

I take a holistic approach and consider the intricate interplay between core strength, pelvic floor health, and overall physical well-being. I've worked with women—from first-time moms to elite athletes—helping them navigate the challenges of prenatal and postpartum fitness.

My expertise extends beyond the clinic. As a mom of two boys and an avid marathoner, I've experienced the same journey that I help others navigate. This blend of professional knowledge and personal experience enables me to offer practical, compassionate advice that goes beyond textbook recommendations.

WHY WE JOINED FORCES

Together, we bring a powerful combination of athletic experience, clinical expertise, and personal insight to your pregnancy fitness journey.

Strong as a Mother was born from our shared belief that pregnant women deserve better guidance—guidance rooted in current research and real-world experience. Whether you're a seasoned athlete or new to fitness, whether this is your first pregnancy or your third, we will meet you where you are.

We believe that every mother deserves to feel strong, confident, and empowered in their pregnancy journey. This book is more than just a guide—it's an invitation to join a community of strong, active mothers. We're here to help you understand what's happening to *your* body, equip you with knowledge, and guide you through safe, effective ways to stay fit and healthy during pregnancy and beyond.

BEYOND EXERCISE

This book takes a holistic approach to pregnancy wellness, recognizing that true strength comes from nurturing your whole self during this transformative time.

PHYSICAL WELL-BEING: We'll guide you through understanding your changing body with scientific insight, covering your body's evolving nutritional needs throughout each trimester, hydration strategies that support both you and your baby, and practical approaches to energy management and recovery that honor your body's demands while maintaining vitality.

MYTH: Incontinence is just part of motherhood

"Get used to leaking—it's just what happens after having babies." How many times have you heard this? While incontinence is incredibly common, should we really accept it as inevitable? We'll take a deep dive into what's happening with your pelvic floor and what you can do about it.

MYTH: There's a right way to give birth

The pressure to have a certain type of birth experience can be overwhelming. But what if the debate between unmedicated and medicated birth is missing the mark? We'll help you understand the full range of birth choices available to you.

MYTH: You should return to exercise postpartum when you feel ready

This vague advice leaves many women wondering what "ready" actually feels like. How do you know if you're doing too much or too little? We'll provide the framework you've been missing.

MYTH: You need to get your body back

The pressure to bounce back after pregnancy is everywhere. But what if the whole concept is flawed? We'll introduce a different way of thinking about your postpartum body.

MYTH: Core work should wait until you're postpartum

"Don't work your core during pregnancy."
"Avoid all ab work."
Sound familiar? The truth about core training during pregnancy might surprise you.

MYTH: Strengthening your pelvic floor will make you susceptible to needing to have a cesarean delivery

Pelvic floor changes facilitate vaginal delivery, and the pelvic floor faces high demands during pregnancy. We'll explore how to keep your pelvic floor strong and flexible for birth.

MYTH: Pregnancy limits athletic potential

Can you maintain your strength during pregnancy? Should you? The latest research challenges traditional thinking and reveals some unexpected insights about exercise during pregnancy.

Myths like these have influenced pregnancy and postpartum guidance for decades, but new research and evolving understanding are revolutionizing how we view pregnancy fitness. Throughout this book, we'll examine these beliefs in detail and provide you with evidence-based information to help you make your own informed decisions.

A NEW UNDERSTANDING OF PREGNANCY WELLNESS

This book isn't just another pregnancy guide—it's a paradigm shift. While many resources focus on your baby's development, we'll help you understand the changes happening in *your body*. This includes learning safe exercise parameters, maintaining core strength, and preventing common issues such as leakage.

Here's what makes our approach different:

- **Tailored Guidance:** We recognize that every pregnancy is unique, and our advice adapts to your changing needs throughout each trimester. (However, keep in mind that it's not meant to replace your physician's guidance.)
- **Empowerment Through Knowledge:** By understanding the reasons behind our recommendations, you'll feel confident in your choices.
- **Focus on Strength:** We'll show you how to build and maintain strength safely during your pregnancy instead of viewing it as a time of limitation.
- **Preparation for Motherhood:** Our approach extends beyond pregnancy to set you up for a stronger postpartum recovery.
- **Expert Perspectives:** You'll benefit from the combined insights of an Olympic athlete and a physical therapist certified in both orthopedics and pelvic health—a unique blend you won't find elsewhere.

REDEFINING PREGNANCY FITNESS

It's time to rethink pregnancy fitness. Gone are the days of vague warnings or unnecessary restrictions. You and your pregnancy journey deserve better than one-size-fits-all advice or outdated limitations. With accurate information and proper guidance, you can embrace an active pregnancy that prepares you for the demands of childbirth and lays the foundation for a confident transition into motherhood.

In the chapters ahead, we'll guide you through each trimester with clear, evidence-based recommendations tailored to your changing body. You'll learn how to work with your body's natural wisdom and build the strength you need for childbirth and beyond. Whether you're an experienced athlete or just beginning your fitness journey, this book will provide the framework to help you thrive during pregnancy.

Remember that your pregnant body isn't fragile—it's powerful and capable of remarkable adaptations. By understanding these changes and learning how to support them, you can approach your pregnancy with confidence instead of caution. Let's empower you with the right knowledge and tools and discover what your body can do.

CHAPTER 2

Understanding Your Core and Pelvic Floor

Before diving into specific exercises or training techniques, it's important to understand the remarkable system at the center of your pregnancy journey: your core. More than just abs, your core is an intricate network of muscles that will adapt to accommodate your baby's growth during pregnancy.

YOUR CORE: MORE THAN JUST ABS

Your core is a complex, cylindrical system of muscles that work together to support your body's movement—allowing you to rotate, bend, and extend. It consists of two main parts: the global core and the deep stabilizing core. Let's take a closer look at the function and importance of each.

Global Core Muscles: Your Body's Outer Support

These are the muscles you can see and feel working:

- The **rectus abdominis** (your six-pack) helps with bending your torso toward your hips or bringing your hips toward your torso. During pregnancy the distance between your rectus abdominus muscles widens to make room for your growing baby. A strong rectus abdominis may help maintain control of this widening. Postpartum, they may play a key role in bringing their distance back together.
- The **obliques** (side abs) assist with rotation and bending to the side. They work with the deep lateral core to provide stability.
- The **erector spinae** (back muscles) help arch your torso backward.
- The hip muscles connected to the pelvis help move the hips in all directions and create stability during single-leg movements.

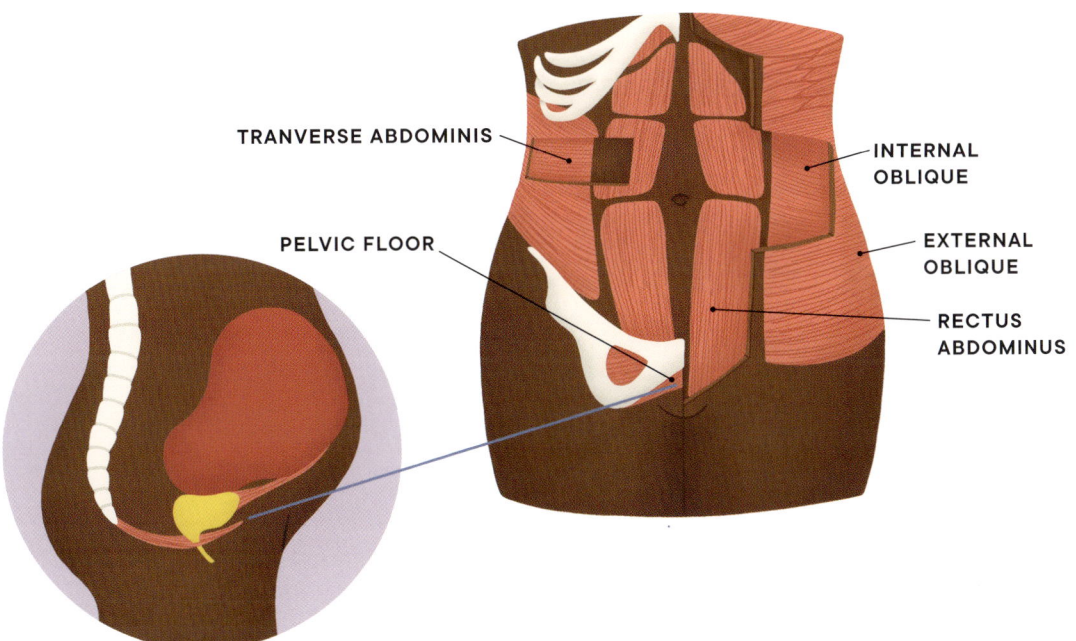

TRANVERSE ABDOMINIS

PELVIC FLOOR

INTERNAL OBLIQUE

EXTERNAL OBLIQUE

RECTUS ABDOMINUS

Deep Stabilizing Core Muscles: Your Internal Support System

Your deep core muscles work behind the scenes to stabilize your entire body:

- The **diaphragm** sits at the top of your core cylinder and is the primary breathing muscle. It can elevate almost two inches during your final trimester and coordinates with your pelvic floor.
- The *transverse abdominis* acts as your body's natural corset or back brace, wrapping around your torso horizontally. It provides deep stability, helps maintain internal pressure, and lengthens as your abdomen creates space for the baby.

- The *multifidi* are small but powerful spinal muscles that control individual *vertebrae* (the bones that make up your spine).
- The **pelvic floor** supports your spine and forms the base of your core cylinder. It holds up your pelvic organs (bladder, uterus, rectum), is crucial for continence and stability, contributes to sexual function and pleasure, and may aid in lymphatic drainage of the pelvis. It undergoes substantial lengthening and stretching during pregnancy and vaginal delivery.
- Although the *rectus abdominis* is considered a global core muscle, it also plays a role in the greater core system during pregnancy. When the fascia (connective tissue) between your six-pack abs isn't as effective, the

rectus abdominis supports the deep and lateral core muscles. It may help reduce abdominal widening (inter-recti distance) and assists in labor contractions, potentially shortening the second stage of labor.

The Connected Core

Your core works as an integrated unit, with each part affecting the others. These connections become especially important during pregnancy and help explain some common experiences: why low back pain often accompanies bladder issues, how abdominal changes can impact pelvic floor function, and why hip pain might indicate pelvic floor challenges. Even your breathing patterns influence core stability, which explains why up to 66 percent of women with diastasis recti experience at least one pelvic floor symptom.

Treating one area alone often isn't enough, and addressing your core holistically often yields better results. Different muscle groups, as well as hormones, ligaments, lifestyle choices, rest, and mental health, all interact and contribute to your overall health, so perfecting one muscle group will not solve all your problems. And remember, while strengthening your core muscles is essential, balance is still key: it is equally vital to ensure that your core can also lengthen and move freely.

The Pelvic Floor: Your Body's Unsung Hero

At the base of your core's muscular cylinder lie the pelvic floor muscles. These muscles are more than just a simple foundation; they're an essential part of your core, and they play various important roles in your body's function and well-being.

Your pelvic floor muscles are true multitaskers. They support your spine and work in harmony with other core muscles to stabilize your entire body as you move. Think of them as a hammock, cradling and supporting your pelvic organs—your bladder, uterus, and rectum. This muscular support, along with the ligaments and fascia, is critical in preventing these organs from prolapsing or descending into the pelvic opening.

But that's not all. Your pelvic floor muscles also guard your continence by supporting the sphincters of your **urethra** (the tube that carries urine from your bladder) and anus. They work tirelessly to prevent unwanted urine or stool leakage, and they're so efficient that you might not even be aware of their constant work!

The influence of your pelvic floor muscles extends to more intimate areas as well, as they play a significant role in the sexual health of people of all genders. These muscles contribute to pleasure and function and are instrumental in achieving orgasm and maintaining erections.

Interestingly, your pelvic floor may even play a part in your body's waste management system, supporting the lymphatic drainage of the pelvic region. Although this function is less understood, it highlights the far-reaching impact of these small but mighty muscles.

A balance of length and strength in the pelvic floor is essential for optimal pelvic health. While strength is vital for many things, problems can arise if the pelvic floor muscles cannot relax and lengthen properly. For instance, occasional urinary leakage can occur when the muscles are too tight, not when they're too weak. An overly tight muscle around the urethra may lack the necessary flexibility to contract effectively, which can impact your ability to stay continent. Signs of an overly tight pelvic floor include constipation, difficulty emptying the bladder, and pain during tampon insertion, vaginal intercourse, or speculum exams.

Your pelvic floor muscles function both automatically and through conscious control. If you aren't experiencing leakage, then your muscles are activating to keep your sphincters closed each time you cough, sneeze, laugh, or move. If you need additional support, you can consciously activate your pelvic floor muscles, just as you would with other muscles in your body.

In the first trimester section, we'll dive even deeper into the pelvic floor muscles. You'll learn techniques and exercises for both contracting to strengthen and relaxing to lengthen them effectively. This knowledge and practice will set you on the path to a healthy, happy pregnancy and beyond.

Understanding Your Changing Core During Pregnancy

Pregnancy and childbirth can have long-term impacts on your core and pelvic floor health, regardless of whether you have a cesarean or vaginal delivery. When your body becomes a home for a baby, hormonal changes affect your muscles, ligaments, and connective tissues in profound ways. Research shows that after pregnancy 50 percent of women will experience changes in the tissues that support their organs and that having a second child increases the risk of prolapse. Interestingly, that risk doesn't increase further after the second pregnancy.

The physical transformation brought about by pregnancy requires a delicate balance between length and strength to achieve optimal pelvic health. Throughout this book, you'll learn exercises that will help create this balance by strengthening the hips, core, and pelvic floor while maintaining the flexibility needed for birth.

Exercise and Inter-Recti Distance

As your body progresses through pregnancy, the rectus abdominis muscles lengthen and change shape to

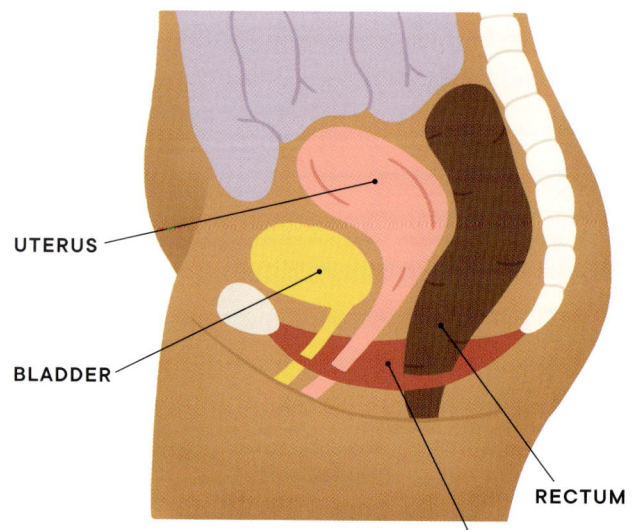

UTERUS

BLADDER

RECTUM

PELVIC FLOOR MUSCLES

accommodate your growing baby. You may notice changes in the appearance of your abdominal muscles, such as a widening gap between the two sides of your rectus abdominis. This increased inter-recti distance is a normal part of pregnancy. In fact, your abdominal muscles may widen significantly during pregnancy, but they often return close to their prepregnancy state postpartum.

Many factors can influence inter-recti distance, such as:

• Hormonal changes
• Collagen levels
• Abdominal muscle strength
• Your body's unique composition
• Your baby's size
• The number of times you've given birth

Maintaining abdominal strength during pregnancy has been shown to control the inter-recti distance and help it rebound afterward. Strong abdominal

muscles provide stability for your abdomen, even as pregnancy hormones alter collagen and reduce muscle fiber tension. In fact, women who participate in sports are less likely to develop a large inter-recti distance.

Many women have been told to avoid abdominal exercises if they notice any increase in their inter-recti distance or a "bulge" on their abdomen. In reality, core exercises are the very thing that can help reduce your inter-recti distance. These exercises should engage both the global core and deep stabilizing core muscles.

Note: If you are someone who is extra mobile—for example, you can bend your body in a unique way or place your hands flat on the ground—and has a higher body mass index (BMI), it's important to pay extra attention to the core exercises in this book.

FROM THE PRO
Jessica's Insights on Inter-Recti Distance

For years, healthcare providers misdiagnosed normal inter-recti distances as *diastasis recti*—an abnormal separation of the abdominal muscles—using the best information they had at the time, which led many women to unnecessarily restrict their core and cardiovascular activities. Today we know better: The natural widening of the rectus abdominis during pregnancy is both normal and necessary.

Although these muscles may not return to their exact prepregnancy distance, this shouldn't limit your activities or cause concern. Unfortunately, outdated knowledge on this topic is so prevalent that many women continue to limit their exercise, feel self-conscious, and seek consultation because they mistakenly assume they have diastasis recti—even when they do not.

When to Seek Support

Current postpartum guidelines suggest that if your abdominal muscles come closer together when you lift your head, you are likely to see improvements. If not, using a gentle belly support binder during the first four to six weeks postpartum may be beneficial in helping you with your daily movements.

While most abdominal changes after pregnancy are normal, consider consulting your healthcare provider if you experience:

- An inter-recti distance of more than 3 centimeters after the fourth trimester
- Persistent low back pain
- Ongoing difficulty lifting

Your Body's Natural Healing Process

Your body has an incredible capacity to heal and recover after pregnancy. As hormone levels shift, they trigger positive changes in your abdominal tissue. Lower levels of estrogen and progesterone help strengthen your abdomen's tensile force by adjusting collagen composition to provide better support. If you're nursing, these changes may occur even faster due to naturally lower estrogen and progesterone levels.

Keep in mind that recovery takes time. Research shows that rebuilding optimal abdominal tone typically takes six to nine months postpartum. During this time, focusing on proper core engagement can help support your body's natural healing process.

LOOKING AHEAD: YOUR PELVIC HEALTH JOURNEY

As we move forward, you'll discover that understanding your core system is just the beginning. In the next chapter we'll explore the myths and realities of pelvic health, addressing common concerns and questions that many pregnant women have but often feel hesitant to discuss. You'll learn that you're not alone in these experiences and, more importantly, that there are evidence-based solutions that can help you maintain strength and confidence throughout your pregnancy journey.

CHAPTER 3

Taking Charge of Your Pelvic Health

Now that you have a better understanding of your core system's anatomy, it's time to explore an often-overlooked but indispensable aspect of pregnancy wellness: pelvic health. Despite affecting people of all ages and in all stages of life, pelvic health issues are often shrouded in silence and misconceptions. It's time to change that narrative.

THE REALITY OF PELVIC FLOOR ISSUES: YOU'RE NOT ALONE

Contrary to popular belief, pelvic floor issues can affect people of all genders and ages, not just those who are pregnant or postpartum. You can experience pelvic floor problems even if you've never been pregnant. For example, if you were a child who struggled with bed-wetting, had accidents when giggling, or experienced constipation, your

YOU'RE NOT ALONE

Because urinary leakage can be hidden with absorbent pads, we often don't realize how many people are dealing with pelvic floor issues. While healthcare providers are working to increase awareness and normalize the symptoms, many women still feel shame or embarrassment around the topic. When it feels difficult to ask for help, refer to these astonishing statistics to remind you that it's okay to do so:

- Half of all women experience pelvic floor changes after delivering a baby.
- When working out, 49.2 percent of women wear leakage protection.
- More than 50 percent of women aged sixty-five or over report urinary incontinence.

pelvic floor may have been the reason. Additionally, athletes of all levels often face pelvic floor challenges due to high-impact activities. Research shows that if you experience leakage during sports early in life, you're more likely to experience it later in life as well.

The first step to healing and strengthening your pelvic floor is knowing that support is available.

Key Fact: Taking care of your pelvic floor can be vital to your health for decades to come. Only about 38 percent of people discuss pelvic floor symptoms with their physician—don't be afraid to speak up!

The Impact on Active Lives

Incontinence is a significant concern for many women and can often be a barrier to regular exercise. This issue goes beyond mere discomfort; it can have a profound impact on overall wellness and quality of life.

Of the 150 minutes of aerobic activity a week that experts recommend, 75 of those should be dedicated to vigorous exercise. Vigorous activity typically involves an intensity level that induces sweating and makes it challenging to have a conversation.

For women who experience leakage, activities such as running, jumping, and other high-impact exercises can feel daunting or even impossible—and the

implications are significant. Research shows that women with severe leakage are 2.6 times more likely to fall short of recommended activity levels. Additionally, 90.3 percent report lowering their exercise intensity, 35.5 percent reduce their exercise frequency, 25.8 percent shorten their exercise duration, 62.7 percent of women who experience leakage take breaks to pee during their workouts, and 80.7 percent avoid certain movements altogether.

By addressing incontinence concerns head-on, you can achieve the intensity, frequency, duration, and work/rest ratio needed to enjoy the numerous benefits of regular exercise. Over the course of a lifetime—from pregnancy and postpartum recovery to peri- and postmenopause—these four factors are essential for supporting health and wellness. They are the key to being strong as a mother.

DEBUNKING PELVIC HEALTH MYTHS: WHAT THE LATEST RESEARCH TELLS US

MYTH: Incontinence is a normal, unavoidable part of motherhood

Birthing a child is a monumental feat for the body. While some women do experience leakage after pregnancy and delivery, it's important to understand that this isn't a *normal* or unavoidable part of motherhood. It's common, yes, but not something we should accept as inevitable.

THE TRUTH ABOUT POSTPARTUM INCONTINENCE

Many women are told that incontinence will resolve once they finish nursing and their hormones return to normal levels. However, hormones alone aren't to blame.

Key Fact: If a woman is experiencing leakage twelve weeks postpartum, she has a 92 percent chance of still facing this issue five years later without intervention. Pelvic floor training is an excellent place to start.

MYTH: Your age, weight, or the number of pregnancies you've had determine the health of your pelvic floor

Many women avoid seeking care for pelvic floor issues due to misconceptions about what causes them. However, contrary to popular belief:

- Family history doesn't determine your fate.
- Weight loss alone isn't a guaranteed solution.
- Age, the number of babies you've delivered, and postmenopausal status do not predict treatment success.

UNDERSTANDING RISK FACTORS

Here are four factors that might impact the success of pelvic floor muscle training:

- Leaking on the first cough
- Experiencing more than two episodes of leakage per day
- Leaking during intercourse
- Leaking immediately after urinating

While these factors can affect your chances of success, pelvic floor training is still worth trying due to its low risk. Your medical team may recommend additional treatment if needed.

THE POWER OF PROFESSIONAL GUIDANCE

The Importance of Early Postpartum Intervention

Pelvic floor training can significantly help reduce leakage in the first year after giving birth, increasing the likelihood that you can return to your preferred form of exercise with less leakage. That said, if you're feeling overwhelmed postpartum or are reading this book later in your recovery, you can still reap the benefits of pelvic floor training no matter when you start. The key is to seek help when you're ready.

Due to hormonal changes, it takes four to six months for your muscles to return to their new resting length after delivery, so be patient with yourself. Engaging in pelvic floor muscle training for a minimum of twelve weeks is the first line of treatment for stress, urge, and mixed (stress and urge) incontinence.

When to Seek Professional Help

A pelvic health specialist can be an invaluable part of your medical team. Consider consulting one if you're experiencing:

- Changes in bowel or bladder habits
- Pain or discomfort
- Issues related to pelvic floor and/or core function

Even if you've been to a pelvic health specialist before, it's worth revisiting, as research and treatment approaches evolve rapidly. For example, we now understand that some degree of pelvic organ movement is normal, even in women who've never given birth.

Here are some reasons to revisit a pelvic health specialist:

- To discuss previously advised activity limitations that were given due to diastasis recti, prolapse, or other conditions
- To ensure your current exercise program is properly tailored to you, with the correct volume and intensity
- To determine if you need to strengthen, lengthen, or relax your pelvic floor

- To identify other factors that might be at play besides muscle function
- To have your healthcare provider measure your vaginal opening to prevent further prolapse
- To evaluate if you're at risk of significant pelvic floor tearing during delivery, even if you haven't given birth before

Working with a pelvic health specialist can help you redefine your movements, activities, and quality of life.

Key Fact: Of the 76 percent of women with a prolapse diagnosis, only 6 percent experience symptoms.

The Effectiveness of Pelvic Floor Muscle Training

Research highlights the following impressive benefits of proper pelvic floor muscle training (PFMT):

- Women are eight times more likely to report being cured or experiencing improvement after twelve weeks of PFMT.
- PFMT leads to significant improvements in quality of life and a reduction in leakage.
- PFMT has no serious adverse effects, making it a low-risk, high-reward treatment.
- For 50 percent of women with stress incontinence, PFMT can be as effective as surgery, but without the associated risks.

Why Professional Help Matters

This book provides comprehensive tools to set you up for success on your pelvic floor journey. If you complete all the exercises in this book and feel that you need further progress, professional supervision can help. To illustrate, home programs that focus solely on pelvic floor exercises have a 17 percent success rate, whereas success rates with professional supervision can range from 60 to 75 percent.

Professionals can prescribe the appropriate exercise volume and intensity for you, identify factors that contribute to pelvic health issues, and guide you on correct technique and positioning. They'll also tailor the program to your specific needs, ensuring your recovery plan supports your individual circumstances and goals.

Common Mistakes to Avoid

A frequent mistake in pelvic floor training is contracting the muscles too strongly. More isn't always better. Contracting the pelvic floor muscles too forcefully can increase pressure on your bladder, and if the sphincter around the urethra isn't strong enough to counteract this pressure, you may experience leakage.

Here's a helpful tip: A half-strength contraction is often more effective than a full-strength one. It allows you to maintain the contraction for longer, doesn't interfere with breathing, and puts less pressure on the bladder. Simple instructions, such as "squeeze your anus," can increase the likelihood of correct performance.

Professional guidance can also help you identify which part of the pelvic floor to focus on to ensure you perform the exercises correctly and effectively.

Key Fact: One in four women cannot perform a pelvic floor contraction correctly using only verbal or written instructions.

Cultural and Personal Perspectives

Our understanding of health is influenced by various factors, including family history, cultural and religious beliefs, societal attitudes about women's health, and access to healthcare information.

While discussing pelvic floor issues may have been taboo in the past, the medical community continues to advance its understanding. Regular check-ins with your healthcare provider can help you stay informed and make the best choices for your body.

LOOKING AHEAD: YOUR PATH TO STRENGTH

In the next chapter, we'll cover exercises and techniques for safely building and maintaining pelvic floor strength during pregnancy. Remember, this journey isn't just about preventing problems—it's about building a strong foundation for pregnancy, birth, and beyond.

CHAPTER 4

Essential Exercise Guidelines

Now that you're familiar with your core system and understand the importance of pelvic health, it's time to put your knowledge into action. In this chapter, we'll explore targeted exercises and foundational techniques to support your pregnancy fitness journey, along with essential safety guidelines to help you exercise confidently and safely.

TAKING CHARGE OF YOUR PELVIC HEALTH

Just as you have agency in labor and delivery—which we'll discuss in detail later in this book—you also have control over your pelvic health. First and foremost, speak up: Don't hesitate to discuss any concerns with your healthcare provider and consider consulting a pelvic health specialist. Now let's begin looking at how to activate your pelvic floor muscles.

PELVIC FLOOR EXERCISES: YOUR FOUNDATION OF STRENGTH

Think back to when we compared your pelvic floor muscles to a hammock that supports your internal organs and controls essential functions. These muscles are vital during pregnancy and childbirth, making them a key focus of your prenatal fitness routine.

As a reminder, your pelvic floor is responsible for:

- Supporting your bones during movement
- Protecting your pelvic organs
- Controlling bladder and bowel function
- Preparing for childbirth
- Facilitating lymphatic drainage
- Contributing to sexual health

Movement is medicine, and exercise is essential for your long-term health. Strengthening your pelvic floor muscles early on can help you stay active and strong.

PELVIC FLOOR EXERCISE 101: HOW TO ACTIVATE YOUR PELVIC FLOOR

The Technique: Static Hold

First, gently tighten the muscles that close your anus, as if you're trying to hold in gas or urine. This activates the levator ani, the posterior pelvic floor muscles that support and lift your organs.

Next, arch your back slightly and focus on contracting the muscles around the clitoris and urethra. This activates the *urogenital triangle*—the anterior pelvic floor muscles—and should feel like you're pulling urine back up into the urethra.

Initially, aim for a 50 percent contraction, held for 3 to 5 seconds, progressing to 33 seconds. Remember, more isn't always better! A 50 percent contraction for 33 seconds is enough to maintain continence. Avoid contracting at 100 percent, as this can create excessive abdominal pressure.

Repeat ten times, three times a day, reducing repetitions as you increase duration. Commit to twelve weeks—the time needed to strengthen muscles effectively.

You'll learn how to coordinate your pelvic floor muscles through the exercises provided in this book. Later, we will take an in-depth look at training these muscles postpartum. In most cases, it's safe to do pelvic floor exercises

BUILDING CONSISTENCY

- Don't let perfection prevent progress.
- Set reminders on your phone to practice.
- Place visual cues around your home.
- Use daily activities as practice prompts.

throughout your pregnancy, and doing so will not change your delivery method. Always consult your healthcare provider if you have any concerns.

PELVIC FLOOR EXERCISES: YOUR FOUNDATION OF STRENGTH

Your pelvic floor muscles contain slow-twitch fibers, which provide endurance and support, and fast-twitch fibers, which enable quick reactions, such as urine control and sexual function. The exercises in this book are designed to target both types of muscle fibers. You'll find the recommended number of repetitions listed at the end of each exercise. If you're not ready to complete the full set or hold for the full duration, gradually work your way up.

Complete instructions for each pelvic exercise can be found in the Exercise Reference Guide on pages 204–205.

Think of these exercises as building blocks—they form the base that supports all your other activities. Whether you're new to exercise or returning to a previous routine, understanding how to move safely while maintaining pelvic floor muscle engagement helps protect your long-term health.

Smart and Safe Strategies for Movement

YOUR PRENATAL WELLNESS PRESCRIPTION

To recap, the American College of Obstetrics and Gynecology (ACOG) recommends:

- Engaging in at least 150 minutes of moderate exercise per week
- Being active on most, if not all, days
- Continuing to move throughout pregnancy, unless there are medical complications

WHEN TO CONSULT YOUR HEALTHCARE PROVIDER

Starting your prenatal fitness journey is exciting, but it's important to get the all clear from your healthcare provider first, especially if you haven't exercised regularly before, have gestational diabetes, or have a BMI outside the recommended range. Don't worry— exercise is generally safe and beneficial, and your healthcare provider can tailor recommendations specific to you.

EXERCISE MODIFICATIONS FOR COMMON CONCERNS

Experiencing leakage during exercise is common during pregnancy. Factors such as a growing uterus, increased amniotic fluid, and pressure on the bladder all contribute to this issue. When combined with the internal pressure from vigorous exercise, the muscles that control the urethra may not be strong enough to prevent leakage.

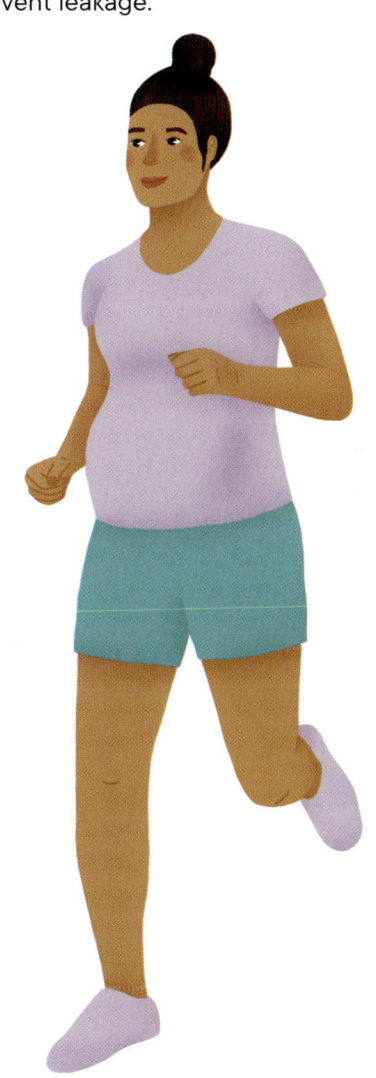

Remember that leakage is a sign to learn more about your body, not a reason to stop exercising altogether. If leakage becomes bothersome, there are several ways to modify your routine to reduce it:

- Switch from standing to seated or reclined exercises.
- Contract your pelvic floor muscles before high-impact movements.
- Exhale during exertion to reduce abdominal pressure.
- Reduce your weights or the intensity of your workout.
- Consider lower-impact alternatives, such as using a stair-climber, elliptical, or rowing machine instead of higher-impact activities (like running).

SAFETY FIRST: UNDERSTANDING EXERCISE CAUTIONS

In some cases, your healthcare provider might advise against exercise. These cases include:

- Ruptured membranes
- Premature labor
- Unexplained, persistent vaginal bleeding
- Placenta previa that persists after twenty-eight weeks of pregnancy
- Preeclampsia
- Incompetent cervix
- Intrauterine growth restriction

- High-order multiples, such as triplets
- Uncontrolled type 1 diabetes, hypertension, or thyroid disease
- Severe anemia
- Serious cardiovascular, respiratory, or systemic disorders

Proceed with caution if you have:
- Recurrent pregnancy loss
- Gestational hypertension
- A history of spontaneous preterm birth
- Mild to moderate cardiovascular or respiratory diseases, such as chronic bronchitis
- Symptomatic anemia or malnutrition
- Eating disorders
- A twin pregnancy (from twenty-eight weeks and beyond)
- A heavy smoking habit
- An extremely high BMI (over 40) or extremely low BMI (less than 12)
- A poorly controlled medical condition, such as diabetes, hypertension, seizure disorders, or hyperthyroidism
- A history of an extremely sedentary lifestyle
- Other significant medical conditions for which exercise is contraindicated

In these cases, it's best to approach exercise with caution or refrain from it altogether if necessary. The most important thing is to consult with your healthcare provider. But don't worry—there are still plenty of ways to stay healthy and prepare for motherhood, which we'll cover in later chapters.

WARNING SIGNS

Stop exercising and contact your healthcare provider if you experience any of the following:

- Chest pain
- Vaginal pain or bleeding
- Regular, painful contractions
- Shortness of breath before or during exercising
- Dizziness or headaches
- Muscle weakness
- Pain or swelling in your calves
- Amniotic fluid leakage

LOOKING AHEAD: BUILDING YOUR ROUTINE

As you begin incorporating these exercises into your daily routine, remember to prioritize consistency over perfection, listen to your body's signals, and adjust the intensity as needed. Contact your healthcare provider if you have any concerns. In the following chapters, we'll discuss trimester-specific guidelines to help you modify these foundational exercises as your pregnancy progresses.

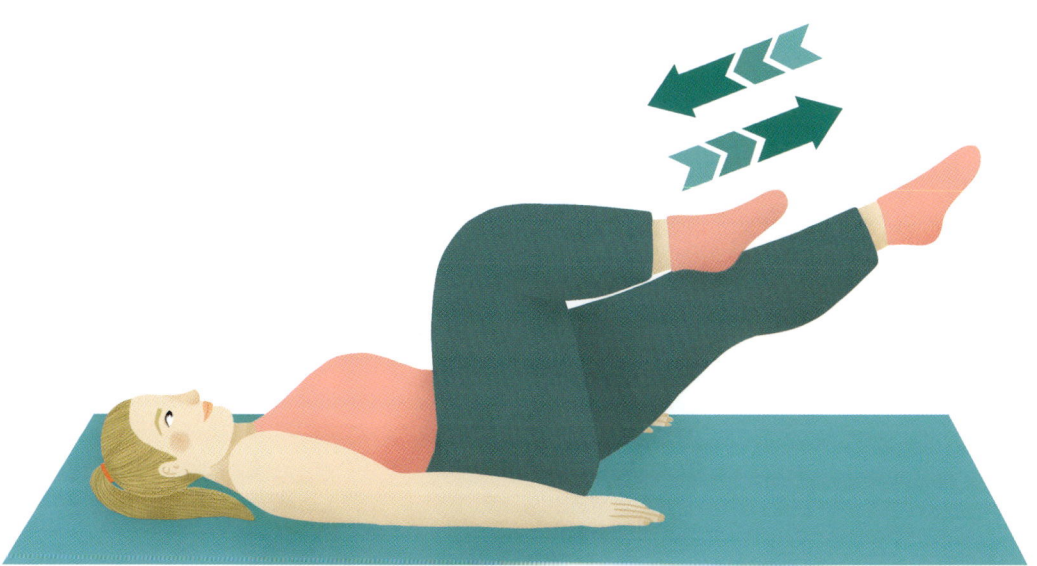

PART II

THE FIRST TRIMESTER

CHAPTER 5

A Time of Rapid Change

Congratulations on your pregnancy! You're at the beginning of an incredible journey that will transform your body, mind, and life. The first trimester is a time of rapid change, often occurring beneath the surface. While you may not look pregnant yet, your body is already working hard to create a new life.

Now that you understand the fundamentals of your core and pelvic floor, it's time to explore how your entire body adapts during these crucial early weeks of pregnancy. This knowledge will help you support your changing body as you begin incorporating the movement principles we've discussed.

In this chapter you'll learn:

- How your body changes week by week and why
- Strategies for managing common symptoms
- Nutrition and hydration guidelines
- How to build your support system
- Tools for emotional well-being

THE IMPORTANCE OF FIRST-TRIMESTER AWARENESS

While many women keep their pregnancies private during the first trimester, understanding what's happening in your body during these weeks is important. Early awareness helps you modify your movement practices as needed, make informed nutrition choices, recognize the differences between normal changes and warning signs, and build habits that support your entire pregnancy.

YOUR BODY'S NEW NORMAL

The first four weeks of pregnancy often pass unnoticed, but your body is already hard at work. Hormone levels begin to rise, and implantation occurs. You might start experiencing early pregnancy symptoms—subtle breast changes, mild fatigue, a heightened sense of smell—although many women feel relatively normal during this time.

During weeks five through eight, changes become more noticeable as your body ramps up support for your growing baby. Your blood volume increases by 30 to 50 percent, and your heart output rises to accommodate the extra blood flow. Your lung capacity expands, and your metabolism shifts significantly as your body prepares to support both you and your baby throughout pregnancy.

Common experiences include changing energy levels, breast tenderness, food aversions or cravings and morning sickness, which can occur at any time of the day despite its name.

As you approach weeks nine through twelve, your body will have nearly reached peak levels of *human chorionic gonadotropin*, the pregnancy hormone responsible for many early pregnancy symptoms. For some women this marks the start of symptom relief, although experiences vary. This phase is often accompanied by shifts in energy levels and the first visible changes to your body. By now, your uterine lining is thickening to support your growing baby—just one of many remarkable adaptations your body makes during pregnancy.

MANAGING FIRST-TRIMESTER EXPERIENCES

Understanding common first-trimester experiences helps you to distinguish between what's normal and when it's time to seek support. We'll outline some typical symptoms below.

Physical Changes

- Extreme fatigue, often peaking around weeks eight to ten
- Nausea or aversions to certain foods
- Lightheadedness
- Food cravings
- Constipation and bloating
- Frequent need to urinate
- Breast changes
- Nasal congestion or occasional nosebleeds
- Changes in your voice

Emotional Shifts

- Fluctuations in mood
- Pregnancy anxiety
- Changes in your sleep pattern

Remember, these symptoms indicate that your body is working hard to support your pregnancy. While they might be uncomfortable, they're often a positive sign and indicate that your hormone levels are rising as they should. Coping strategies vary from person to person, so staying in touch with your healthcare providers is key.

Balancing Energy, Nourishment, and Activity

Your first trimester requires the right balance to maintain energy levels that support both you and your baby. Understanding this balance helps you maintain appropriate activity levels, support your baby's development, manage fatigue, and prevent energy deficiency.

Warning signs of energy imbalance, also known as relative energy deficiency in sport (RED-S), include:

- Constant fatigue that does not get better with rest
- Slower than usual recovery from physical activities
- Feeling weaker during exercise or movement
- Frequent illnesses
- Bone injuries
- Persistently feeling down, depressed, or irritable
- Difficulty concentrating
- Low iron levels
- Digestive issues
- Sleep disturbances

Monitoring Your Energy Balance

As you now know, maintaining proper energy balance is important during both pregnancy and postpartum, especially if you have an active lifestyle. It ensures you're meeting the needs of your changing body, supporting your baby's growth, and fueling your physical activities.

Remember that your energy needs can change throughout your pregnancy and postpartum. Regular check-ins with your healthcare provider and a registered dietitian can help ensure you're meeting your energy needs.

ENERGY CHECK-IN

Each week, take a moment to assess your:
- Overall energy levels (on a scale of 1 to 10)
- Sleep quality (on a scale of 1 to 10)
- Hunger patterns
- Exercise recovery time
- Mood
- Concentration level

Next, make necessary adjustments, such as:
- Adding nutritious snacks between meals
- Modifying your activity level
- Ensuring you're getting enough rest

Hydration: A Pregnancy Essential

Maintaining your energy balance goes beyond proper nutrition; it also requires adequate hydration. Drinking enough water during pregnancy supports your baby's development and your body's needs. By staying hydrated you help your body:

- Maintain healthy amniotic fluid levels
- Digest, which reduces constipation
- Eliminate waste from your body
- Absorb water-soluble vitamins (especially B vitamins) from your prenatal supplements
- Circulate nutrients
- Produce energy
- Build and maintain muscles
- Regulate your body temperature

You can determine your personal hydration needs by taking your current body weight in pounds, dividing that number by 2 to get your base need in ounces, then adding 8 to 10 ounces as your pregnancy bonus.

   For example, if you weigh 150 pounds, your base need would be 75 ounces of water. Including your pregnancy bonus (8 to 10 ounces), your total daily water intake goal should be 83 to 85 ounces.

Hydration Markers

New research suggests that your fluid intake may be less indicative of your hydration levels than how often and how much you urinate, which can vary based on your activity level. If you experience urinary symptoms—such as peeing too often, too infrequently, or feeling intense urges to urinate—you may need to reassess your hydration needs or seek healthcare consultation.

TIPS FOR STAYING HYDRATED

Start these habits early on in your pregnancy:

- Carry a reusable water bottle wherever you go.
- Infuse water with natural flavors like lemon or lime.
- Set regular reminders to drink.
- Track your water intake using a bottle with marked measurements, a hydration tracking app, or your pregnancy journal.

While most of your fluid intake should consist of water, all liquids count! This includes soup, coffee, tea, some fruits—and yes, even your celebratory glass of champagne postpartum.

Important Reminder

Urine color is typically a good indication of hydration status but can be affected by prenatal vitamins. It's a good idea to focus on reaching your daily water goal based on your activity and monitoring your hydration markers rather than relying solely on monitoring urine color.

Smart Nutrition Strategies

Pregnancy changes how your body processes carbohydrates, making regular snacking more important than ever. Think of your nutrition as a continuous process rather than three distinct meals. Your growing baby needs a steady stream of nutrients, and frequent small meals can help manage nausea and maintain stable blood sugar levels.

Pre-exercise snacks help ensure you have the energy needed for movement, while post-exercise nutrition supports recovery. During longer workout sessions, having a light snack every 45 minutes can help maintain your energy levels. Add about 300 extra calories to your daily diet to support your pregnancy, focusing on nutrient-dense foods that provide a mix of carbohydrates, proteins, and healthy fats.

SNACK IDEAS

Here are some snack ideas for you to try:

- **Pre-Exercise:** Energy bars, dried fruit, crackers with nut butter
- **During Exercise:** Energy chews, small pieces of fruit
- **Post-Exercise:** Greek yogurt with berries, chocolate milk, hummus with vegetables

MAKE A PERSONALIZED SNACK PLAN

Using your pregnancy journal, list five to ten easy-to-prepare snacks that you enjoy and that meet your nutritional needs. Consider factors such as portability, preparation time, and nutrient balance. Keep this list handy for quick reference when planning your meals and workouts.

Remember to consult your healthcare provider about your specific nutritional needs during pregnancy.

Emotional Wellness and Support

The first trimester isn't just physically challenging—it can be an emotional rollercoaster as well. Your emotional journey deserves as much attention as your physical one. During your first trimester, you might feel excited and anxious at the same time, experience uncertainty about the changes ahead, worry about keeping the pregnancy private, or need to process a changing sense of identity. These feelings are completely normal as you navigate this transformative time.

Building Your Village

Think of your pregnancy support system as a community built specifically for your needs. At its center are the healthcare providers who will guide you through pregnancy and birth.

Your core healthcare team might include:

- Obstetrician
- Gynecologist
- General practitioner
- Naturopathic physician
- Pelvic health specialist
- Mental health professional
- Midwife or doula
- Registered dietician

Note: We'll cover additional healthcare practitioners who may be worth adding to your care team later in the book.

TRACKING YOUR EMOTIONAL WELL-BEING

Monitoring your emotional well-being is just as important as tracking your physical health during pregnancy and postpartum. Each week, take a moment to reflect on your overall mood and describe it in a few words. Then, rate the following aspects on a scale of 1–10:

1. Energy levels
2. Sleep quality
3. Stress levels
4. Motivation for daily activities
5. Enjoyment of usual activities

Remember that it's normal to experience a range of emotions both during pregnancy and postpartum. The goal of mood tracking is not to judge your feelings but to increase self-awareness and ensure you're getting the support you need. If you're consistently scoring low or notice concerning trends over the course of several weeks, consider seeking additional support from your healthcare provider or a mental health professional.

Beyond this core team, consider the various types of support you'll need, such as emotional encouragement, practical help, and guidance from those who have walked this path before. To help identify the support you might need at different stages of your pregnancy journey and postpartum experience, ask yourself:

- What support do I need this week?
- Who can provide this support?
- What barriers might prevent me from asking for help?
- How can I overcome these barriers?

Your village might include people you haven't met yet, such as fellow parents in a prenatal class or members of a pregnancy support group. Building and nurturing these connections during your pregnancy can create a strong support system for when your baby arrives. Don't be afraid to reach out and let others know you value their support. Many people are happy to help, but they may not know how unless you ask.

While you don't need to assemble your entire support network right away, knowing your options can help you feel more prepared and supported.

Understanding these foundational aspects of your first trimester will help prepare you for safe and effective movement. In the next chapter, we'll look at first-trimester exercise guidelines and modifications.

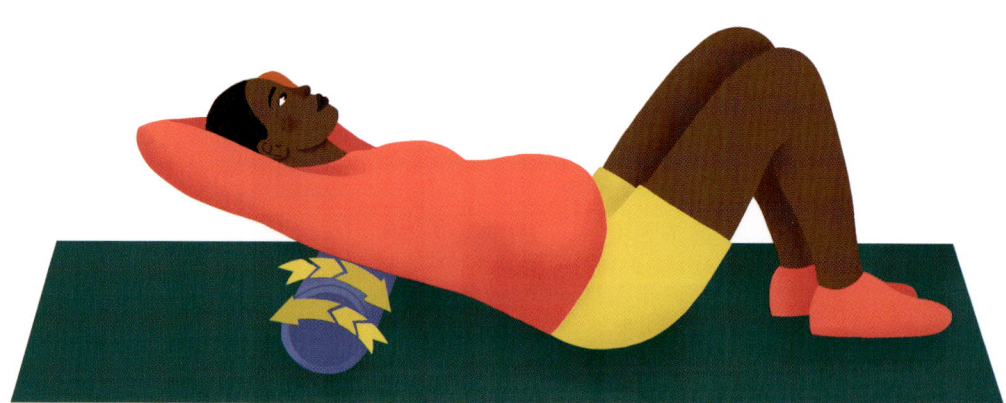

CHAPTER 6

Your Prenatal Fitness Tool Kit

Now that you understand how your body changes during the first trimester, let's dive into some safe and effective exercise strategies for your pregnancy. This chapter will equip you with fundamental tools and concepts to guide your movement journey throughout all three trimesters.

BUILDING A ROUTINE THAT WORKS FOR YOU

Consistency is key in prenatal fitness, and the secret to being consistent is doing what you love. Whether you find joy in dancing, walking, or swimming, choose activities that make movement feel like a natural part of your day rather than a chore.

If you're looking to replace high-intensity activities or start a new routine, consider these safe activities to get your heart rate up. Anything in the "Modified Activities" list should be done with caution and only if comfortable.

Low-Impact Options

- Walking
- Swimming
- Stationary cycling
- Elliptical exercise

Group Activities

- Dancing
- Low-impact aerobics
- Prenatal yoga

Modified Activities

- Rowing
- Stair climbing
- Prenatal kickboxing

ACTIVITY SELECTION

To select activities that are right for you, ask yourself the following questions:

- Does this activity bring me joy?
- Is it easy to modify when needed?
- Do I feel confident doing it?

Safety Note: Most activities are safe, and you can often continue many of your usual exercises. However, avoid scuba diving and water skiing. Consult your physician for balance-dependent activities such as gymnastics, horseback riding, skiing, and ice skating. After your sixteenth week of pregnancy, be cautious with activities that pose a risk of abdominal impact, as blunt force trauma to the belly could harm your baby. Consult your physician about outdoor activities at elevations above six thousand feet to ensure optimal oxygen supply, as well as activities like hot pilates or yoga, where overheating may occur.

Modify Your Fitness Routine to Your Changing Body

If you've been active before pregnancy, you shouldn't need to make significant changes during the first trimester. That said, it's important to pay attention to how your body feels after a workout to ensure that the volume and intensity are right for you. If you experience pain or discomfort lasting more than one hour after exercising, need an afternoon nap, or wake up feeling tired or sore, follow these steps to adjust your workout intensity:

- Add rest cycles: For running, try alternating between running and walking until you reach your desired distance.

For biking, split your session into two 20-minute sets instead of one continuous 40-minute workout.
- If you're still more tired than usual, reduce the volume or intensity by 10 to 20 percent. Remember, you can continue exercising at a lower rate.
- If fatigue, pain, or discomfort persist, switch to lower-impact activities. Opt for gentler activities like walking, which raises your heart rate and can help guide the baby down the birth canal in the final weeks of your pregnancy.

Stop exercising immediately if you feel faint, lightheaded, or nauseous at any point. Additionally, remember to:

- **Stay Cool and Hydrated:** Your body's temperature and hydration needs are changing.
- **Ensure Good Ventilation:** When exercising indoors, use a fan to circulate the air.
- **Time Your Workouts Wisely:** If you live in a warm climate, exercise early in the morning or late in the evening to avoid peak temperatures.
- **Be Mindful of Changes to Your Breathing:** Progesterone stimulates your lungs to "over-breathe," providing more oxygen for you and your baby.

Note: Due to increased blood volume, your heart rate can increase by 10 to 20 beats per minute during pregnancy.

That increase can affect how you feel, particularly during more intensive workouts, and is an important factor to consider when calculating your heart rate, which we'll explore below.

Understanding Exercise Intensity

Monitoring your exercise intensity during pregnancy is key to staying safe and getting the most out of your workouts. We'll now explore several methods to help you find and maintain the ideal level of exertion for you.

Checking Your Heart Rate

Monitoring your heart rate helps you track exercise intensity. If you don't have a wearable device that tracks your heart rate, you can manually check it at these pulse points:

YOUR WRIST: With your palm up, place your index and middle fingers on the inside of your wrist, just below the base of your thumb.

YOUR NECK: Place your index and middle fingers on your neck, just beside your windpipe.

Start from zero when you feel the first pulse, counting your heartbeats for 30 seconds. Then multiply by two to find your beats per minute (bpm).

Practice checking your heart rate first thing in the morning (before getting out of bed), during moderate exercise, and during your cooldown.

Key Fact: Heart rate isn't the most reliable indicator during pregnancy. It is helpful to compare your heart rate to your talk test, which we'll discuss below, to understand the intensity ranges that are right for your body.

Calculate Your Maximum Heart Rate

To determine your maximum heart rate (MHR), you can use this formula:

220—your age = your MHR

Calculate Your Target Heart Rate

Your target heart rate is a percentage of your MHR. While it's not a perfect metric, it can be a useful tool. Pregnancy can affect the accuracy of using heart rate as a gauge, but knowing your target heart rate can still be helpful, especially if you use a smartwatch to monitor your workouts.

Use the following calculations to find your target heart rate range:

- **Lower limit (64 percent of MHR):** MHR × 0.64
- **Upper limit (76 percent of MHR):** MHR × 0.76

Your ideal workout intensity falls between these two numbers.

Remember, during your first trimester, your resting heart rate may be higher due to increased blood volume. Factors such as hydration, fitness level, and the type of exercise you're doing can also affect your heart rate. Use the target heart rate range as a guide, but make sure to always listen to your body. You can also use an exertion scale to assess your workout intensity.

Mastering the Talk Test

The talk test is one of the most reliable ways to gauge exercise intensity during pregnancy. Here's how it works:

- **Light Intensity:** You can sing or speak in full sentences with ease. This level is ideal for warming up or on days when you prefer gentler movement.
- **Moderate Intensity:** You can speak one or two sentences but notice some heavier breathing. This is the ideal intensity level for most workouts and should be your target.
- **Vigorous Intensity:** You can only say a few words at a time. If you experience this during pregnancy, it's time to lower your workout intensity.

Try this: During your next workout, practice the talk test by reciting a nursery rhyme or singing your favorite song. Pay attention to how your breathing changes as you increase or decrease your intensity and record your experiences to track your progress over time.

Calculate Your Exertion Scale

The Borg rating of perceived exertion (RPE) scale is a tool that helps you determine your workout intensity on a scale from 6 to 20. Think of 6 as sitting quietly and 20 as the hardest effort possible. Here's how to identify which number you're at:

- **Very Light Effort (6–8):** You can hold a conversation easily, and your breathing is normal.
- **Light Effort (9–11):** You're comfortable talking, but your breathing is slightly elevated.
- **Somewhat Hard (12–14):** You can talk but not sing, and your breathing is more noticeable.
- **Hard (15–17):** You can only say short phrases, and your breathing is quite heavy.
- **Very Hard (18–20):** You're having a hard time speaking, and your breathing is very heavy.

During pregnancy, aim to stay in the 12 to 14 range, in which you're working hard but can still hold a conversation. At this level:

- Your breathing should be noticeable but not labored.
- You should be able to speak in complete sentences.

- You should be working hard but remain in control.
- You should feel slightly warm but not overheated.

This moderate intensity aligns perfectly with both the talk test and safe heart rate zones for pregnancy. If you can't talk comfortably, ease back. If you can sing easily, consider increasing your intensity slightly, provided you feel comfortable doing so.

Essential Exercise Components

It might be tempting to jump straight into your workout and then rush off as soon as you're done, but understanding how to begin and end your exercise sessions properly is especially important during pregnancy. Let's look at these key components to make every workout safer and more effective.

Warm-Up and Cool-Down

Proper warm-up and cool-down routines are vital during pregnancy. When you first conceive, your blood vessels relax, and your body starts retaining more water and salt to increase blood plasma volume. This can sometimes lead to symptoms such as fatigue, a racing pulse, nausea, pallor, sweating, or dizziness.

A proper warm-up and cool-down can help manage blood pressure changes, reduce the risk of varicose veins, prevent dizziness, support temperature regulation, and improve workout quality.

YOUR WARM-UP GUIDE

Start with:
- Gentle walking
- Light jogging in place

Transition to mobility and activation exercises:
- Controlled squats
- Arm circles
- Shoulder rolls
- Activation exercises on pages 36–37

Finish with:
- Pelvic tilts
- Gentle back stretches

YOUR COOL-DOWN GUIDE

Start with:
- Gradually decreasing pace
- Slowing your breathing to a normal rate

Transition to:
- Gentle stretching
- Major muscle group work

Finish with:
- Deep breathing
- Pelvic floor relaxation

Try this: Design your personal warm-up and cool-down routines, aiming for at least 8 to 10 minutes for each, and experiment with different activities to find what feels best for your body. You can also use this time to practice mind-fulness or set intentions for both your workout and your day. And don't forget: A pregnancy journal can help you keep track of which warm-up and cool-down activities work best for you throughout all stages of your pregnancy.

Body Maintenance: Balancing Flexibility and Activation

As your pregnancy progresses and your baby grows, your body undergoes significant changes that impact your posture. These changes include your back muscles tightening and your adductors becoming tighter as well. Your pelvis begins tipping forward while your hip muscles start shortening to accommodate your growing belly. Additionally, your lower body bears increasingly more weight, which significantly increases the demands placed on your knees, hips, ankles, and arches throughout your pregnancy journey.

The following exercises are designed to balance stretching with strengthening, helping you maintain comfort and stability throughout these changes. Aim to perform these exercises at least three times per week, although daily practice can offer additional benefits. Each session combines gentle stretching with targeted strengthening moves.

Essential Flexibility Work

Here is a list of recommended stretches. You can find detailed instructions and recommendations for each exercise in the Exercise Reference Guide. If your main goal is to improve flexibility, be sure to check out the exercises in the third-trimester section.

- **Child's Pose Stretch:** Opens your back while protecting your sacroiliac joint
- **Dynamic Adductor Stretch:** Releases tight inner thigh muscles
- **Side-Lying Rotation Stretch:** Maintains hip and back mobility
- **Calf Stretch/Bent Knee Calf Stretch:** Supports comfort in the ankles and feet
- **Standing Quadriceps Stretch:** Releases tight front hip muscles
- **Standing Snow Angels:** Opens the chest and the sides of your body

Essential Activation Work

Some areas of the body require activation (targeted muscle engagement) in addition to stretching, as they can start feeling tight due to the postural changes and increased demands that pregnancy places on them.

- **Seated Pelvic Tilts on Ball:** Engages your core and pelvic floor
- **Arch Lifts:** Strengthens foot stability
- **Calf Raises:** Activates the lower leg muscles

- **Bent-Knee Calf Raises:** Deepens calf muscle support
- **Seated Leg Curls (Banded):** Maintains back knee stability
- **Seated Leg Extensions (Banded):** Maintains front knee stability
- **Side Steps (Banded):** Integrates full-body control

These exercises, along with many others in this book, will help support your changing posture.

With these fundamental tools in place, you're ready to begin your first-trimester exercise introduction. In the next chapter, we'll cover weekly exercises designed to support and benefit your body.

SMART ADAPTATION WHEN DISCOMFORT ARISES

Sometimes pain—rather than intensity—can limit your workouts. If you're experiencing pain, seek clearance from your healthcare provider. However, if you're dealing with discomfort rather than pain, consider the following steps:

- Ensure the discomfort is exercise-related.
- Stop if the pain increases by 3 or more points on a scale of 1–10.
- Monitor your post-workout recovery.
- Adjust the intensity or impact level if post-workout discomfort persists for more than one hour after the workout.
- Consider alternative, lower-impact activities.

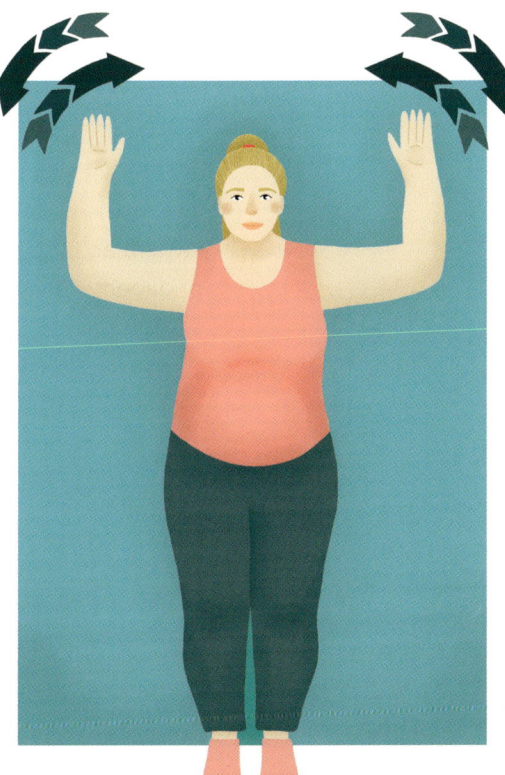

STANDING
SNOW ANGELS

Gwen Jorgensen

Olympic gold medalist

After winning gold in triathlon at the 2016 Olympics, I wanted to start a family but wasn't sure how that would impact me as an athlete. There was limited information about exercising during pregnancy, especially for elite athletes, and I was uncertain about how to train safely. I knew I needed fitness for my body, my baby, and my mental health.

My body became my guide throughout my first pregnancy, teaching me to adapt and listen. The first trimester surprised me with how little I could do—I felt sick constantly and had to drastically cut back on actual training. Instead of fighting these changes, I focused on getting outside daily. Some days I managed a run, but more often I walked, which helped tremendously with my nausea and reminded me that movement didn't have to be intense to be beneficial.

In the second and third trimesters, my energy returned and I could train about two hours daily, swimming, biking, and running. During my first pregnancy, swimming felt awful, so I mostly ran and biked. I ran over 100 miles weekly and did structured workouts, though my pace had changed significantly. Before pregnancy, I ran mile repeats under 4:45; while pregnant, those same repeats were 6:00–6:30 pace. I loved that I could still challenge myself without focusing on times, instead prioritizing what made my body and mind feel strong. Staying hydrated and cool during all workouts became essential.

My second pregnancy taught me that each experience is unique. Swimming felt wonderful, so I spent more time in the pool and less running. Working with pelvic floor physical therapist Jessica Dorrington and other experts guided me through both pregnancies and postpartum recovery. I learned crucial lessons, including that my pelvic floor was too tight and that doing pelvic floor strengthening exercises may not benefit me, but rather hinder my progress.

The key to mental and physical health during pregnancy is listening to your body and being patient with yourself as you navigate these profound changes.

CHAPTER 7

Your First-Trimester Exercise Program

Your first trimester is the perfect time to establish exercise habits that will benefit you throughout your pregnancy and postpartum recovery. The foundational exercises we'll introduce in this chapter are carefully designed to support your changing body. By the time you reach the fourth trimester, these exercises will also support your return to fitness.

Each week you'll learn new movements designed to progress with your changing body. These exercises will help you build a strong foundation throughout your pregnancy while mastering proper form that will serve you well beyond birth. By becoming familiar with each movement during pregnancy, you'll have the confidence and muscle memory needed to safely return to these exercises during your postpartum recovery journey.

FOR EVERY BODY

If you're new to exercise, welcome! Research shows that starting a safe exercise routine during pregnancy can benefit both you and your baby. Always consult your healthcare provider for clearance first.

For experienced exercisers, the movements in this book are designed to complement your current routine. While you may choose to continue your regular workouts with appropriate modifications, incorporating three to four of these pregnancy-specific exercises will help support your changing body.

Think of these exercises as an investment in your postpartum recovery. In each week, you will find several variations to meet your ability level. Choose the variations that best match your fitness.

Before beginning any exercise, it's essential to understand proper form and starting positions. For detailed instructions on:

- Core engagement techniques
- Basic starting positions (lying, seated, standing, etc.)
- Form reminders and breathing techniques

See the Exercise Fundamentals on page 199.

FIRST-TRIMESTER EXERCISE INTRODUCTIONS: WEEKS ONE TO TWELVE

During the first four weeks, we will focus on teaching you how to activate your core stabilizing muscles—your body's foundation. These fundamental movements support all the activities you do during and after pregnancy. While you might not often think about your abdominal muscles—particularly your rectus abdominis—during pregnancy, research shows that maintaining their strength could help shorten the pushing phase of labor. Your abdominal muscles work continuously as your belly expands and may assist you during delivery. Think of core training as preparation for one of your body's most athletic moments: bringing your baby into the world.

After focusing on the core stabilizing muscles, you'll progress to more advanced movements that engage your supporting muscles. These first weeks feature more challenging exercises because your body will have fewer pregnancy-induced limitations. The goal is to master these core-strengthening exercises early in pregnancy, before shifting your focus to the hip, knee, and calf muscles. Once you reach the third trimester, mobility and stretching take precedence.

Note: If you are starting this program as a newcomer to exercise, choose the exercises that feel comfortable for your fitness level and form as you move through the weeks, using the week numbers as a guide rather than an absolute.

For exercises with different levels (beginner, intermediate, advanced), start with the version that fits your ability and advance as appropriate. Aim to select three or four exercises per week to build consistency and strength.

WEEK ONE: Core Foundations

During this first week, you'll build the control center for all your future movements. We'll focus on activating your core muscles and establishing proper breathing patterns—fundamental skills that will support your body during pregnancy.

EXERCISE	SETS × REPS	PAGE
Breathing	2-3 minutes	199
Core Engagement Holds	5 secs × 5 reps, 2 sets	215
Sit to Stand	10 reps, 2 sets	250

WELLNESS INSIGHT
If you're new to exercise, that's great! Starting now can benefit both you and your baby. Remember to check in with your healthcare provider before starting.

FREQUENCY
Daily

WEEK TWO: Adding Arm Movement

Now that you've built your core foundation, we'll challenge it by adding arm movements. This week we'll introduce weights (kettle-bells or free weights) to further enhance your core control. Think of each arm movement as an opportunity to maintain a strong foundation while managing additional forces. This combination of core stability and arm movement will help prepare you for daily activities that involve reaching, lifting, and carrying. Remember to choose weights that allow you to maintain proper form throughout each set, as technique should always take priority over the amount of weight you're lifting.

EXERCISE	SETS × REPS	PAGE
Core Engagement Holds	5 secs × 8 reps, 2 sets	215
Arm Lifts	10 reps per side, 2 sets	207

WELLNESS INSIGHT
Your heart is already working harder, as it's pumping 30–50 percent more blood than before you were pregnant.

EQUIPMENT
• 4-6 lb weights or filled water bottles (optional)
• Mat

FREQUENCY
3 days per week

WEEK THREE: Leg Integration

EQUIPMENT
• Mat

FREQUENCY
3 days per week

This week marks an important progression as you begin to coordinate your core strength with leg movements. Practicing these movement patterns now will help prepare your body to maintain stability, so you can move with confidence throughout your pregnancy journey—whether you're navigating stairs, picking up objects, or simply keeping your balance during daily activities.

EXERCISE	SETS × REPS	PAGE
Heel Slides	10 reps per side, 2 sets	223
Knee Fall Outs	10 reps per side, 2 sets	224
Knee Straighteners	10 reps per side, 2 sets	226
Leg Lifts	10 reps per side, 2 sets	228
Marches	10 reps per side, 2 sets	230

WEEK FOUR: Adding Movement

EQUIPMENT
• Loop band
• Chair

FREQUENCY
3 days per week

This week we'll introduce a versatile tool to enhance your workout: resistance bands. We'll work with two types: loop bands for targeted muscle work and long resistance bands anchored to a solid surface for more dynamic movements. Resistance bands provide feedback on your movement quality while helping you build strength and stability, allowing you to increase difficulty while maintaining control.

LEVEL	EXERCISE	SETS × REPS	PAGE
Beginner	Marches	10 reps per side, 2 sets	230
Intermediate	Seated Marches	10 reps per side, 1-2 sets	237
Advanced	Seated Marches (Banded)	10 reps per side, 1-2 sets	238

WEEK FIVE: Building Hip Strength

Your hips and glutes play an important role in maintaining a stable core during pregnancy. This week we'll focus on exercises designed to strengthen these muscle groups while reinforcing core control: bridge movements. As your pregnancy progresses and your center of gravity shifts, strong hips and glutes help you stay balanced, reduce strain on your back, and support everyday activities such as climbing stairs or getting up from a chair.

LEVEL	EXERCISE	SETS × REPS	PAGE
Beginner	Bridges	10 reps, 1-2 sets	212
Intermediate	Bridges with Heel Lifts	10 reps per side, 1-2 sets	213
Advanced	70/30 Bridges	10 reps per side, 1-2 sets	206

WELLNESS INSIGHT
Strong abdominal muscles help prevent back pain and support digestive health.

EQUIPMENT
• Mat

FREQUENCY
3 days per week

WEEK SIX: Advanced Hip Work

Now that you've started building hip strength, we'll add some complexity. Building on last week's exercises, which helped you develop refined hip control and stability, these advanced movements will prepare your body for the increasing demands of carrying your growing baby. Progress only if you have mastered the previous exercises.

LEVEL	EXERCISE	SETS × REPS	PAGE
Beginner	Single-Leg Bridges	10 reps per side, 1-2 sets	246
Intermediate	Single-Leg Bridges (Weighted)	10 reps per side, 1-2 sets	246
Advanced	Hip Thrusters	10 reps, 1-2 sets	223

EQUIPMENT
• Light weights (for weighted variation)
• Bench or jump box (for hip thrusters)
• Mat

FREQUENCY
3 days per week

WEEK SEVEN: Core Progression

EQUIPMENT
• Long resistance band (for banded variation)
• Mat

FREQUENCY
3 days per week

Congratulations! You've built your foundation, and your core muscles are now ready for the next challenge: controlled resistance training. Think of this progression as layering your strength. We'll add resistance thoughtfully while maintaining the proper form you've already mastered. This approach will help your core develop the endurance and strength needed to support your growing belly while protecting your back and pelvic floor.

LEVEL	EXERCISE	SETS × REPS	PAGE
Beginner	Core Curl Ups	10 reps, 1-2 sets	214
Intermediate	Core Curl Ups (Banded)	10 reps, 1-2 sets	215

WEEK EIGHT: Coordination and Control

EQUIPMENT
• Mat

FREQUENCY
3 days per week

This week you'll work on your coordination and learn how to keep your core connected and engaged while you move.

LEVEL	EXERCISE	SETS × REPS	PAGE
Beginner	Low Bicycle	10 reps per side, 1-2 sets	229
Intermediate	Toe Taps	10 reps per side, 1-2 sets	257
Advanced	Runner's Toe Taps	10 reps per side, 1-2 sets	235

WEEK NINE: Side–Body Strength

As part of your core, the muscles along the sides of your body help support your growing belly and maintain balance, providing stability for your pelvis during single-leg activities and help prevent back strain. Strengthening them now will prepare you for the increasing physical demands of carrying your baby throughout your pregnancy. Choose the appropriate exercise for your ability.

LEVEL	EXERCISE	SETS × REPS	PAGE
Beginner	Kneeling Side Plank	30 seconds, 2 sets per side	227
Intermediate	Side Plank	30 seconds, 2 sets per side	243
Advanced	Side Plank Leg Lifts	10 reps per side, 1-2 sets	243

WELLNESS INSIGHT Did you know that getting less than 8 hours of sleep per night increases your risk of injury? Sleep is an essential part of your wellness routine, so be sure to listen to your body and rest when you need to.

EQUIPMENT
• Exercise mat recommended

FREQUENCY
3 days per week

WEEK TEN: Hip and Core Stability

This week we'll focus on movements that help maintain hip strength and ensure proper alignment as your pregnancy progresses. This will become especially important later in your pregnancy when your stance naturally widens to accommodate your growing belly, and your center of gravity shifts forward.

LEVEL	EXERCISE	SETS × REPS	PAGE
Beginner	Kneeling Side Plank Hip Drops	10 reps per side, 1-2 sets	227
Intermediate	Kneeling Side Plank Hip Drops with Leg Lift	10 reps per side, 1-2 sets	228
Advanced	Side Plank Hip Drops	10 reps per side, 1-2 sets	243

WELLNESS INSIGHT Remember that your body is changing. Allow yourself plenty of time to adapt to new routines.

EQUIPMENT
• Loop band (optional)
• Exercise mat recommended

FREQUENCY
3 days per week

WEEK ELEVEN: Full Body Integration

WELLNESS INSIGHT
It is recommended to eat at least every 4 hours to maintain energy. Plan your snacks around your workout times, and pack them in your purse or gym bag so they are readily available.

EQUIPMENT
• Exercise mat recommended

FREQUENCY
3 days per week

This week we'll combine strength work with coordinated, full-body movements. We'll focus on activating the multifidi—deep muscles that help stabilize the spine. When functioning well, the multifidi help you move smoothly during daily activities that require twisting or turning, like vacuuming and getting in and out of the car. Spinal stability is especially important in sports and activities that involve pelvic rotation, as it ensures efficient movement while protecting your back.

LEVEL	EXERCISE	SETS × REPS	PAGE
Beginner	Bear Plank Knee Taps	10 reps per side, 1-2 sets	208
Intermediate	Bear Plank Leg Lifts	10 reps per side, 1-2 sets	209
Advanced	Full Plank	30 seconds, 1-2 sets	221

WEEK TWELVE: Dynamic Movement

WELLNESS INSIGHT
Your body is adapting to support your growing baby. Be attentive to your body's signals for rest and recovery needs.

EQUIPMENT
• Loop band
• Agility ladder or tape/markers to create a pattern

FREQUENCY
3 days per week

During this final week of your first trimester, we'll introduce exercises that teach your body to move dynamically and with control. These agility-focused exercises will help you master movements—such as quick directional changes and controlled transitions—that build on your current strength and stability. Learning these now will prepare you to modify them as needed in later trimesters.

LEVEL	EXERCISE	SETS × REPS	PAGE
Beginner	Jump Prep	8 reps, 2 sets	224
Intermediate	Hops (Banded)	8 reps, 2 sets	224
Advanced	Ladder In/Outs	8 reps, 2 sets	228

Five Tips for Learning Your Strong as a Mother Exercises

MASTER THE FUNDAMENTALS FIRST

- Perfect basic core engagement before advancing.
- Return to the fundamentals whenever your form starts to waver.

FOCUS ON THE THREE CS: CORE, CONTROL, AND CONNECTION

- Maintain core engagement and alignment during all movements.
- Control every phase of each exercise.
- Stay connected to your breath and your body's signals.

PROGRESS AT YOUR OWN PACE

- Master your current level before advancing to the next one.
- Incorporate three to five exercises into your existing routine.
- Prioritize quality over quantity.

TRACK YOUR JOURNEY

- Identify the best time of day for your workouts.
- Write down exercises that feel particularly good or challenging.
- Record modifications that work for you.
- Monitor your energy levels before and after workouts.

LISTEN TO YOUR CHANGING BODY

- Remember that some days will feel easier than others.
- Adjust the intensity based on your current energy level.
- Stop if something feels off.
- Celebrate what your body can do.

LOOKING AHEAD

Congratulations! You've now built a solid foundation. The exercises, wellness strategies, and self-awareness you've developed will empower you as you move into your second trimester.

During this next phase of your pregnancy, your energy will likely increase, and early pregnancy symptoms may ease, giving you the perfect opportunity to build on the foundational skills you've developed so far. The strength and body awareness you've cultivated will help support you as more visible body changes occur.

Keep your first-trimester pregnancy journal entries handy—they'll provide valuable insights into your body's patterns and preferences as you progress. Remember that each phase of pregnancy brings opportunities for being aware of, and tuning in to, your body's ever-evolving needs. You've learned to listen to your body; now you'll discover new ways to work with it as your pregnancy progresses.

Take a moment to celebrate completing the first phase of your pregnancy journey. Then turn the page to discover how we'll build on the skills you've learned so far as you enter your second trimester.

PART III

THE SECOND TRIMESTER

CHAPTER 8

Finding Your Stride

Welcome to your second trimester! Often called the honeymoon phase of pregnancy, this stage usually brings a surge of new energy and relief from early symptoms. As your body settles into pregnancy, you'll discover new opportunities to build strength and stay active, all while learning to adapt to your changing shape and shifting center of gravity.

YOUR BODY'S NEW NORMAL

Your body has done something remarkable: It has created a stable environment for your growing baby. As the challenging symptoms of early pregnancy ease, you'll have the chance to focus on building strength and enjoying movement in new ways. This trimester will allow you—and your body—to find a new rhythm.

Understanding Weight Changes

The weight gain, which may have been minimal or even challenging if you experienced nausea during your first trimester, now typically follows a more predictable pattern. This weight gain isn't just about the numbers on a scale; it's your body building vital resources for both you and your baby, making this process not only natural but necessary. Your body is supporting the growth of your baby and placenta while also increasing the volume of your amniotic fluid, blood, and plasma. All of these changes contribute to healthy weight gain.

You may have gained roughly 1 to 4 pounds in your first trimester. During the second trimester, you can expect to gain about 0.5 to 1 pound per week, although this amount can vary based on your starting weight and the number of babies you're carrying. For instance, if you're pregnant with multiples, you can typically expect to gain between 37 to 54 pounds.

Your healthcare provider will help you determine your ideal weight gain based on your prepregnancy weight, overall health factors, whether you're carrying multiples, and your specific pregnancy needs.

It's important to focus on gradual, steady weight gain rather than rapid fluctuations. Your healthcare provider will monitor your weight throughout your pregnancy to ensure that both you and your baby stay healthy. Remember that this book contains general guidelines. Your healthcare provider can provide personalized recommendations based on your specific situation.

When it comes to movement, keep in mind that the extra weight puts more strain on your knees, ankles, and feet—especially on the inside of your arch and midfoot. You might also experience more frequent cramps in your feet and legs, as your calves work harder to support the additional weight you now carry in front of your center of gravity.

YOUR CHANGING SYSTEMS

Cardiovascular Adaptations

During this trimester your body reaches peak efficiency, resulting in your:

- Heart output increasing by 40 to 50 percent
- Blood volume continuing to expand
- Heart stroke volume rising by 15 to 25 percent
- Kidney blood flow improving, leading to more frequent urination
- Heat regulation improving due to increased blood flow

Muscular Changes

As your baby grows, certain muscle groups need extra attention because your:

- Back muscles work harder to maintain posture
- Core muscles lengthen to support your growing belly
- Pelvic floor muscles handle increasing pressure
- Calves manage the additional weight in front of your center of gravity

Hormonal Laxity Changes

During pregnancy and into the fourth trimester, your body will be affected by hormonal changes. The placenta dramatically increases levels of estrogen and progesterone, which, in turn, increase joint mobility throughout the fourth trimester—contrary to the popular belief that relaxin is solely responsible for these changes.

BALANCE ADJUSTMENTS

Your balance changes significantly during pregnancy. Pregnant women are more than twice as likely to fall as those who aren't pregnant, so it's important to incorporate exercises into your routine that help you maintain balance. The single-leg exercises in this book are an excellent place to start.

Here are some of the main ways in which your body adapts to help you maintain balance during pregnancy:

- Your stance widens to prevent falls.
- Your side-to-side movement increases while walking.
- Your forward motion requires more conscious effort.
- Your muscles work harder to maintain stability as joint mobility increases.

It's important to note that your baby is no longer protected by the pelvis after the first trimester. Continue prioritizing balance exercises, and carefully consider the risks and benefits of activities that could lead to falls.

POSTURAL SHIFTS

Try: Stand sideways in front of a mirror and observe your posture, noticing how your body naturally adjusts to balance your growing belly. Understanding these changes helps you work with them rather than against them.

Purposeful adjustments to your posture are as your body shifts to accommodate your growing baby. While these changes might feel considerable, remember that many of them will naturally reverse after pregnancy.

EXERCISE ROUTINE: BALANCE

Try these balance exercises to improve your stability:

- Single-Leg Squats at Wall
- Single-Leg Squats
- Single-Leg Squats to Runner's Drive
- Single-Leg Hops (Side-to-Side)
- Single-Leg Hops (Forward/Backward)
- Glute Wall Reach
- Runner's Clamshells
- Side Step Downs
- Front Step Downs
- Single-Leg Balance
- Single-Leg Balance Clock Reaches
- Runner's Balance Challenges

Please find detailed instructions for each exercise in the Exercise Reference Guide. You can do these exercises all at once or spread them out throughout the day or week, depending on what works best for you. No matter how you choose to incorporate them into your routine, they will help strengthen the connection between your muscles and brain.

Upper Body

As your belly grows, your upper body compensates by:

- Shifting backward for balance (which may cause you to round your shoulders and jut your chin forward)
- Creating space (your ribs may rise upward by as much as two inches during pregnancy, possibly resulting in hand numbness)
- Broadening your chest (which increases its circumference)

Lower Body

The increased weight also affects your lower body in the following ways:

- Your back and hip muscles naturally shorten, along with your adductors.
- Your knees, hips, ankles, and foot arches take on additional pressure.
- Your calf muscles manage increasing demands, which may cause cramping.
- Your foot arches may flatten.
- Your feet may lengthen, widen, and increase in volume.

Pelvis

Your pelvis begins tilting forward, which can:

- Increase pressure on the lower back joints
- Change the position of your *sacrum* (the keystone of your pelvis)
- Increase pressure on the front areas of your hips
- Affect your walking and running patterns

FROM THE PRO
Jessica's Insights on Pelvic Health During the Second Trimester

Your second trimester brings rapid changes to your body and pelvic floor. The pelvic floor muscles are now working overtime to stabilize your pelvis, support your growing uterus and other organs, and manage bowel and bladder control. At the same time, pregnancy hormones are preparing these muscles to lengthen and soften in preparation for birth—a remarkable but challenging process.

You might experience changes in bladder control, especially during exercise, or reduced sensation during intercourse. Increased pelvic pressure, along with occasional difficulty controlling gas or bowel movements, can also become noticeable.

The work you do during pregnancy directly impacts your postpartum recovery. Many women ask about starting pelvic floor exercises after birth, but the most successful approach is to maintain strength throughout pregnancy, similar to exercise. Think of it as building your foundation; every time you exercise now will contribute to better function later.

Keys to Success

Pay attention to how different exercises affect your pelvic floor.

- Modify activities if you notice any discomfort (heaviness, pain, or aches in the pelvis).
- Be consistent with your pelvic floor exercises.
- Engage your entire core during moderate lifting activities.
- Listen to your body's signals for rest or modification.

Remember, these changes are both normal and purposeful. Your body is preparing for birth while maintaining strength—a delicate balance that the exercise program in this book will help you achieve.

Managing Common Challenges

Understanding and managing pregnancy-related swelling, aches, and pains requires attention and strategy. While increased blood volume and fluid retention play important roles during pregnancy, they can also lead to challenges that need to be actively addressed.

Debunking Round Ligament Pain Myths

MYTH: The pain around the pelvis is round ligament pain

Round ligament pain is a common yet often misunderstood aspect of pregnancy. Many people assume that any abdominal pain is likely round ligament pain, but why is this particular ligament so troublesome?

The Truth About Round Ligament Pain

During pregnancy your uterus stretches significantly. Between your twelfth and sixteenth weeks, it transitions from being a pelvic organ to an abdominal one. By your twentieth week, it can be felt at your belly button, and by the thirty-sixth week, your uterus—which was once nestled in your pelvis—extends up under your ribs.

Round ligament pain affects 10 to 30 of pregnant women and typically manifests as a cramp-like discomfort in the lower abdomen. The pain may radiate to the groin and is more common if you've been pregnant before. Round ligament pain can be sharp when you move suddenly and sometimes radiates to the front of the pubis or feels like a tugging sensation in the vagina. This type of pain generally occurs at the beginning of the second trimester, coinciding with a period of rapid uterine growth, uterine wall thickening, and blood vessel expansion.

However, it's important to note that not all abdominal discomfort during pregnancy is due to round ligament pain. There are several potential causes of new abdominal pain, including Braxton Hicks contractions and your baby's movements.

Abdominal pain can also signal more serious conditions, such as an ectopic pregnancy or uterine rupture, HELLP syndrome, placental abruption, and acute fatty liver. Because these conditions can be serious, it's crucial not to dismiss all abdominal pain as round ligament pain. Always consult your healthcare team about new symptoms to ensure proper diagnosis and care.

If your healthcare provider determines that you're experiencing round ligament pain, you may benefit from the following strategies to help ease your discomfort:

- Wear an elastic belly band or use dynamic taping to support your belly.
- Focus on strengthening the stabilizing core muscles mentioned throughout this book.
- Consider gently stretching your abdomen.
- Try gently massaging the outer genital area and pubic mound.
- Lie on your side, supporting your belly with pillows.
- Support your belly when sneezing, coughing, or laughing by holding it or bending forward slightly.
- Take a warm bath to relax your muscles.
- Avoid positions, postures, and activities that increase your pain.
- Move slower, especially when changing positions.

Remember, while these techniques can help manage round ligament pain, it's important to keep your healthcare provider informed about any symptoms and changes that you experience.

Swelling and Circulation

During pregnancy your body produces about 50 percent more blood and body fluids to support your growing baby. While some swelling (also known as edema) is normal, particularly in your feet, ankles, and hands, you can take proactive steps to manage it effectively. Let's look at a multi-faceted approach that can help you manage edema during your pregnancy.

MOVEMENT IS MEDICINE

Regular activity keeps your circulation flowing, much like a proper cool-down after training. Try the following techniques:

- Go for a daily walk at a comfortable pace.
- Swim or exercise in the water (bonus: the water pressure helps reduce swelling).
- Do simple foot and ankle exercises throughout the day.
- Create a gentle stretching routine.

REST WITH PURPOSE

Strategic rest is as important as movement. Consider these strategies:

- Elevate your feet above your heart when resting.

- Lie on your side, particularly your left side, to promote optimal blood flow.
- Use pillows to support your body during sleep. For example, you can place a pillow between your knees to support your hips or under your belly when sleeping on your side.
- Take short breaks during long periods of standing or sitting.

RECOVERY TECHNIQUES

The following recovery techniques may help alleviate swelling and discomfort:

- Massage swollen areas, gently moving from distal areas toward your heart, to help reduce fluid retention.
- Try a prenatal massage with a qualified therapist.
- Apply cool compresses to swollen areas.
- Consider regular pool sessions for natural compression that helps reduce swelling.

COMPRESSION SUPPORT

If you're expecting a long day, you may benefit from wearing graduated compression socks. Make sure they're made from comfortable, breathable materials, and put them on first thing in the morning, before swelling builds.

FOOTWEAR

Good footwear promotes blood circulation, which can help reduce swelling. When selecting shoes, choose ones with good arch support and adjustable closures made from breathable materials to account for changes in length, width, and volume of your feet.

TIPS FOR BETTER CIRCULATION

- Keep a pair of compression socks in your workout bag.
- Set hydration reminders on your phone.
- Do ankle and foot exercises when seated.
- Create a bedtime elevation routine.
- Track your most effective management strategies.

While swelling is normal, these signs warrant immediate attention:

- Sudden or severe swelling
- Uneven swelling, with one leg significantly more swollen than the other
- Swelling in the face or hands
- Significant changes in swelling patterns

Supporting Your Changing Body

DAILY ESSENTIALS

Paying attention to your food and water intake becomes increasingly important throughout your pregnancy to manage swelling. Here are some tips for your second trimester.

DAILY FLUID NEEDS

- Revisit your hydration needs on page 27.
- Monitor the color of your urine (light yellow indicates good hydration, but keep in mind that prenatal vitamins can alter the color of your urine).

NUTRITIONAL ADJUSTMENTS

- Minimize your intake of processed, high-sodium foods.
- Focus on potassium-rich foods, such as bananas and sweet potatoes.
- Moderate your caffeine intake.
- Choose nutrient-dense, hydrating foods, such as watermelon and cucumber.

MONITORING YOUR BODY'S SIGNALS

In your pregnancy journal, track:

- Times of day when the swelling increases
- Activities that help reduce swelling
- Effective rest positions
- Your hydration levels and their effects on your body

As you've now learned, your second trimester brings significant changes to your body's structures, systems, and needs. By understanding these changes, you can move safely and effectively during this important phase. In the next chapter we'll explore how to apply this knowledge through specific exercises and movement patterns designed to support your strength as your baby grows.

Kate Grace

Olympic finalist, 2x national champion,
4x national team member

My biggest concern about maintaining fitness during pregnancy was ensuring I did everything to keep my baby healthy. With so much contradictory information available—and most advice framed in the negative like 'don't get too hot, don't lift too heavy, don't go too hard'—I was genuinely confused about what I could safely do. Jessica and my doctors were instrumental in assuring me that exercise wasn't just okay, it was actually beneficial for both my baby and me. They gave me the confidence to understand that I didn't have to choose between my athletic dreams and my desire to start a family.

What surprised me most was how good I felt during pregnancy, especially as I moved into the second trimester. While I experienced fatigue in the first trimester, I discovered that exercise actually helped with nausea, and that appropriate strength work helped me avoid feeling uncomfortable as my body changed to carry my growing baby.

I was amazed by my body's ability to adapt while still maintaining athletic performance.

As an Olympian ranked third in the world when I became pregnant, I was at the peak of my career and had been training at an international level for ten years. My typical routine included running about ten times per week with varying intensities—usually two hard sessions, two moderate efforts, and six easy runs—plus three days of strength training and physical therapy. I made the decision to get pregnant at that time because I wanted to compete at the 2024 Olympic Trials.

During my first and second trimesters, I maintained my normal training schedule with important modifications. I kept the ten weekly runs and three lifting sessions but strategically cut out the hardest workouts, focusing instead on moderate and threshold efforts. This approach made sense because you typically only need the most intense workouts closer to racing season, and I obviously had time before competing again.

I made one significant change during the hottest part of summer in my first trimester: I stopped my weekly long runs to ensure I could stay properly hydrated and cool. I replaced them with mile repeats, taking enough rest between each repetition to drink water and check in with how I was feeling. This modification allowed me to maintain fitness while respecting my body's changing needs.

The most important lesson I learned was that I could do far more than I initially thought possible while pregnant. The key was truly learning to listen to my body—I never pushed through pain or intense discomfort, and I paid careful attention to how I felt in the day or two following workouts to ensure I was responding well to training.

I did learn one lesson the hard way when I didn't follow Jessica's advice about lifting modifications. I ended up injuring my SI joint doing a heavy deadlift, which taught me to respect how ligaments change composition as the body prepares for birth. It's simply not worth pushing over the line with lifts if it means injuring yourself and having to take time off.

During my third trimester, I really pulled back on workout intensity because that felt right in my body. I still exercised seven days a week, but it was mostly easy intensity. Running became increasingly uncomfortable, so I shifted to uphill walking and elliptical work while continuing lighter strength training.

Setting time goals—like working out for an hour daily—rather than focusing on pace or specific activities worked best for me.

My return to sport had some unexpected challenges, including what we believe was a hip labrum injury during labor, which slowed my timeline. I started with very short walk-runs at six to seven weeks but didn't attempt full runs until after twelve weeks. Looking back, I wish I had treated the entire twelve to eighteen months as 'postpartum' and maintained a more structured progression plan instead of reverting to normal training too quickly.

Having support from experts like Jessica was crucial in making me feel confident and excited about my pregnancy journey—both as a new mom and as an athlete. I loved learning that having a baby could actually improve my athletic experience.

My advice to other athletes: find experts who affirm that being active benefits both you and your baby. Don't focus on times—you will slow down, but the work matters and will benefit you for years to come. More than ever, I was amazed by what my body could accomplish. If I could carry, birth, and feed a baby, I felt like I could do anything.

CHAPTER 9

Your Second-Trimester Exercise Program

EMBRACING MOVEMENT IN YOUR HONEYMOON PHASE

The second trimester is the perfect time to shift your mindset toward supportive movements that will help prepare you for the journey ahead.

A New Approach to Movement

During this trimester you'll focus on the duration of your activity rather than distance or pace, tune in to your body's daily needs, and adapt your activities based on your comfort level. Remember that modifications reflect wisdom, not weakness.

EXERCISE OPTIONS FOR YOUR CHANGING BODY

Many women find that they need to modify their usual activities during the second trimester. This isn't a step backward—it's a smart adaptation to your body's changing needs. If higher-impact activities become uncomfortable, consider:

- Power walking, especially uphill
- Prenatal yoga or stretching classes
- Stationary bike or elliptical machine workouts
- Modified strength training

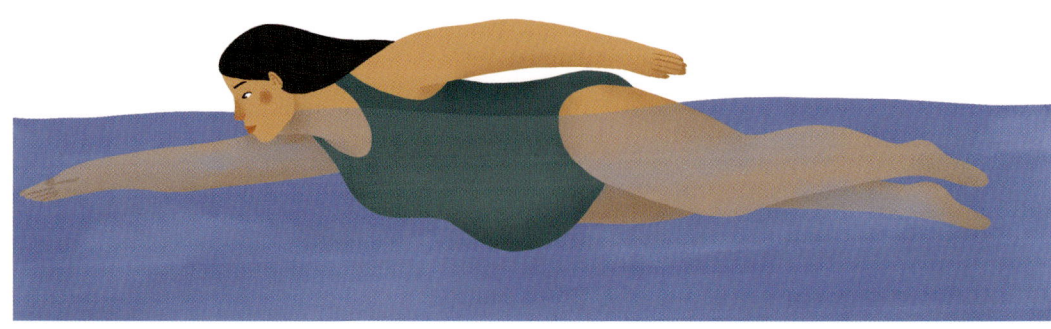

In addition, exercising in water is beneficial in many ways. It:

- Offers natural resistance without stressing your joints
- Supports your body as you exercise to reduce added weight
- Helps regulate your temperature during your workout
- Helps reduce swelling in the legs and feet
- Enhances your mood and energy levels

Note: Always consult your healthcare provider before starting or continuing any exercise program during pregnancy. They can provide personalized advice tailored to your health and the progression of your pregnancy.

WATER WORKOUT OPTIONS TO TRY

- Aqua jogging (consider using a flotation belt and/or shoes)
- Swimming laps
- Taking water aerobics classes
- Walking
- Pool-based stretching exercises

Setting Yourself Up for Success

Before starting your exercise program, make sure your equipment provides the support you need. Let's look at some essentials.

EXERCISE GEAR ESSENTIALS

Properly Fitting Sports Bras: Breast tissue contains delicate collagen fibers that can easily be strained. As hormonal changes increase your breast size early in your pregnancy, ensuring proper support is crucial. Here are some important considerations:

- Opt for straps that are at least two fingerbreadths wide.
- Test the bra's support by jumping; your breasts should shift only minimally.
- Consider wearing two bras for added support, but ensure they don't restrict your breathing.

Properly Fitting Footwear: During pregnancy your feet may widen, lengthen, flatten, or swell due to extra fluid, weight, and hormonal changes. For many women, this can equate to ½ to 1 size difference. Keep these recommendations in mind to ensure your footwear provides the right support:

- Account for potential changes in your arches.
- Allow for adjustments in both width and length.
- Perform the insole test (see next page).
- Ensure there is adequate room for your toes to balance and push off.

Note: Don't forget—your old shoes can still be useful. Consider donating them to organizations that repurpose shoes or to local resources for those in need of clothing.

THE INSOLE TEST

Take out the insole of your shoe and stand on it. If your toes extend past the top or spill over the sides, you may need a larger size or a wider toe box.

Why is this important? Because your toes need room to wiggle, as this allows them to function both as a flexible system for balance and a rigid system for push-off and strength.

PREPARING FOR YOUR EXERCISE PROGRAM

As you begin your second-trimester exercise program, keep these key principles in mind:

PRIORITIZE COMFORT: Rather than focusing on maintaining prepregnancy abilities, tune into what feels supportive each day. Your body's needs may be changing on a day-to-day basis.

BALANCE THROUGH MOVEMENT: Strengthening and stretching exercises should be key components of your routine. This dual approach helps maintain muscle tone, promotes flexibility, and reduces discomfort.

MIND YOUR PELVIC FLOOR: With increased blood flow to your kidneys, you will produce more urine. Hormonal changes may allow your bladder to store more urine as well. However, if your pelvic floor muscles or urethra can't close effectively, you may experience more leakage. If leakage becomes bothersome, consider switching to lower-impact exercises or modifying your positions. Also, keep in mind that nighttime bathroom visits are normal during pregnancy.

TARGET KEY AREAS: To support your changing body, focus on exercises that strengthen your knees, hips, back, and core. This targeted approach helps maintain stability and reduces the risk of discomfort or injury.

LIFTING TECHNIQUES IN YOUR SECOND TRIMESTER

As your pregnancy progresses, lifting requires a more mindful approach. With your belly growing and your spine changing shape, it's important to adapt how you manage everyday lifting tasks. During pregnancy the space between your vertebrae decreases, and the natural curve of your back becomes more pronounced. Combined with your growing belly, these changes affect how you can lift and move objects safely.

Safe Lifting Guidelines

Focus on these key principles when lifting:

- Use your leg strength rather than your back muscles.

- Keep your feet shoulder-width apart and your knees slightly bent.
- Keep your spine neutral.
- Engage your entire core.
- Avoid twisting while lifting.
- Reduce the load for overhead and floor-level lifts.
- Don't use your legs to push furniture if you're experiencing pelvic discomfort.
- Aim for a weight you can lift for 12 to 14 repetitions, 1 to 2 sets.

Listening to Your Body's Signals

Your tolerance for lifting depends on several factors, including your pelvic floor function, ligament condition, bladder position, intra-abdominal pressure response, and strength training experience. These elements work together to determine what feels safe for your changing body.

You should modify your approach or consult a pelvic health specialist for personalized guidance if you experience concerning symptoms such as urine or stool leakage, a sensation of heaviness in your pelvic region, or discomfort during or after lifting sessions.

Remember that the goal is to maintain functionality while protecting your changing body. When in doubt about any activity or if experiencing persistent symptoms, seek help or consult your healthcare provider to discuss your individual needs.

SECOND TRIMESTER STRENGTH PROGRESSION: *Weeks Thirteen to Twenty-Six*

Just like in the first trimester, the exercises during this phase build progressively, focusing on developing strength through squats, jumps, lunges, and other lower-body workouts—all while maintaining proper core engagement.

Always listen to your body and consult your healthcare provider before starting a new exercise regimen. If you experience any pain, discuss it with your healthcare provider or pelvic health specialist. Modifying your activities can often help alleviate pain and keep you active.

Note: Remember to revisit the basic instructions for all exercise starting positions in the Exercise Reference Guide. Maintaining proper form and technique is essential.

SUPPORTING YOUR BABY'S GROWTH THROUGH EXERCISE

The placentas of healthy women who exercise regularly grow faster and function more efficiently than those of women who are healthy but do not exercise regularly. This increased efficiency results in a better supply of oxygen and nutrients for your baby. Aim to exercise most, if not all, days of the week, striving for a weekly total of 150 minutes of moderate-intensity activity.

WEEK THIRTEEN: Plyometric Foundations

WELLNESS INSIGHT
As you move into your second trimester, now is the perfect time to take advantage of your—likely increasing—energy levels while being mindful of your changing balance.

EQUIPMENT
• Tape or markers to create a target square (optional)

FREQUENCY
2–3 days per week

This week we'll focus on learning safe plyometric patterns. These controlled jumping exercises help maintain lower-body strength and power while teaching proper landing mechanics. Review the form and technique to familiarize yourself with exercises beyond your current ability and consult your medical provider for safe high-level activity.

Note: Position two two-foot pieces of tape on the floor, crossing them at right angles to form a plus sign with four quadrants as reference points for jumps.

LEVEL	EXERCISE	SETS × REPS	PAGE
Beginner	Double-Leg Hops (Forward/Backward)	8 reps, 2 sets	216
Beginner	Double-Leg Hops (Side-to-Side)	8 reps, 2 sets	217
Intermediate	Single-Leg Hops (Forward/Backward)	8 reps, 2 sets	247
Intermediate	Single-Leg Hops (Side-to-Side)	8 reps, 2 sets	247

WEEK FOURTEEN: Advanced Plyometrics

EQUIPMENT
• Low jump box or step

FREQUENCY
2–3 days per week

This week we'll introduce more dynamic jumping patterns, which challenge your stability and control.

LEVEL	EXERCISE	SETS × REPS	PAGE
Beginner	Scissor Jumps	8 reps, 2 sets	235
Intermediate	Box Jumps	8 reps, 2 sets	211
Advanced	Box Taps	8 reps per side, 2 sets	212

WEEK FIFTEEN: Squat Foundations

Squats are excellent for building lower body strength and stability. This week we'll focus on proper squat mechanics and core integration.

LEVEL	EXERCISE	SETS × REPS	PAGE
Beginner	Mini Squats	10 reps, 1-2 sets	230
Intermediate	Medium Squats	10 reps, 1-2 sets	230
Advanced	Full Squats	10 reps, 1-2 sets	230

WELLNESS INSIGHT
Your uterus is gradually becoming an abdominal organ. Consider using supportive gear, such as a maternity support belt, for added comfort during activities.

EQUIPMENT
• Weights (optional)

FREQUENCY
3 days per week

WEEK SIXTEEN: Advanced Squat Variations

This week we'll challenge your stability and strength through unilateral movements.

The exercises below use the Mini Squat as a reference. Adjust the depth of your squat or add weight to increase the difficulty. For all exercises this week, only attempt a squatting or lunging depth that allows you to maintain proper form, ensuring your arches stay lifted with your knees aligned over your feet.

LEVEL	EXERCISE	SETS × REPS	PAGE
Beginner	70/30 Squats	10 reps per side, 1-2 sets	207
Intermediate	Single-Leg Squats at Wall	10 reps per side, 1-2 sets	248
Intermediate	Single-Leg Squats	10 reps per side, 1-2 sets	248
Advanced	Single-Leg Squats to Runner's Drive	10 reps per side, 1-2 sets	248

WELLNESS INSIGHT
As your uterus shifts into the abdominal cavity, you may notice less urgency to pee and less leakage compared to your first trimester.

EQUIPMENT
• Weights (optional)

FREQUENCY
2–3 days per week

WEEK SEVENTEEN: Lunge Progressions

EQUIPMENT
• Weights (optional)

FREQUENCY
2–3 days per week

This week we'll focus on controlled lunge variations to enhance single-leg stability and hip strength, while ensuring proper form to protect your knees and hips.

LEVEL	EXERCISE	SETS × REPS	PAGE
Intermediate	Forward Lunges	10 reps per side, 1-2 sets	218
Intermediate	Side Lunges	10 reps per side, 1-2 sets	242

WEEK EIGHTEEN: Calf Strength Foundations

WELLNESS INSIGHT
Reading to your baby in utero is valuable. Consider reading the remainder of this book out loud.

EQUIPMENT
• Stable surface for support
• Weights (optional)

FREQUENCY
3 days per week

As your pregnancy progresses, your calves require extra attention to help support your growing weight and shifting balance. Focusing on calf-strengthening exercises now will benefit you during the third trimester.

Note: It's important to maintain a lifted arch and grounded toe during both the elevation and lowering phases of calf raises to build foot strength and ensure proper movement.

LEVEL	EXERCISE	SETS × REPS	PAGE
Beginner	Arch Lifts	20 reps, 1-2 sets	207
Beginner	Calf Raises	10 reps, 1-2 sets	213
Intermediate	70/30 Calf Raises	10 reps per side, 1-2 sets	206
Advanced	Single-Leg Calf Raises	10 reps per side, 1-2 sets	247

WEEK NINETEEN: Advanced Calf Series

Building on last week's exercises, we'll introduce bent-knee variations to target different aspects of calf strength.

Note: Maintaining a lifted arch and grounded toe during both the elevation and lowering of calf raises is important for your foot strength and proper movement.

LEVEL	EXERCISE	SETS × REPS	PAGE
Beginner	Bent-Knee Calf Raises	20 reps, 1-2 sets	210
Intermediate	Bent-Knee 70/30 Calf Raises	20 reps per side, 1-2 sets	209
Advanced	Bent-Knee Single-Leg Calf Raises	20 reps per side, 1-2 sets	211

WELLNESS INSIGHT
Changes in your belly are happening more quickly now. Consider taking a weekly belly photo to track and celebrate your baby's growth.

EQUIPMENT
• Chair
• Weights (optional)

FREQUENCY
3 days per week

WEEK TWENTY: Standing Calf Control

This week we'll focus on strengthening the deeper calf muscles to support good posture and balance during daily activities.

LEVEL	EXERCISE	SETS × REPS	PAGE
Beginner	Runner's Bent-Knee Calf Raises	20 reps per side, 1-2 sets	233
Intermediate	Runner's Bent-Knee Calf Raises (Weighted)	20 reps per side, 1-2 sets	233

EQUIPMENT
• Chair
• Weights (optional)

FREQUENCY
3 days per week

WEEK TWENTY-ONE: Inner Thigh Strength

WELLNESS INSIGHT
Try adding uphill power walks to your routine, as they keep your heart rate elevated and provide a great workout with minimal impact.

This week you'll strengthen your inner thigh muscles, which help stabilize your pelvis during pregnancy.

Note: Keep your standing knee soft, avoid leaning sideways, and use fingertip support as needed for the following exercises, especially as pregnancy shifts your center of balance.

EQUIPMENT
- Chair
- Stable surface for support
- Long resistance band

FREQUENCY
2–3 days per week

LEVEL	EXERCISE	SETS × REPS	PAGE
Beginner	Seated Hip Adduction	10 reps, 1–2 sets	236
Intermediate	Standing Hip Adduction	10 reps per side, 1–2 sets	253
Advanced	Standing Hip Adduction (Banded)	10 reps per side, 1–2 sets	253

WEEK TWENTY-TWO: Balance and Stability

WELLNESS INSIGHT
Your body is creating a new life. If you're feeling tired, remember that sometimes a nap can be more powerful than a workout.

This week's exercises will challenge your balance while strengthening your inner thigh muscles.

EQUIPMENT
- Wall
- Jump box or sturdy raised surface
- Mat

FREQUENCY
3 days per week

LEVEL	EXERCISE	SETS × REPS	PAGE
Beginner	Wall Copenhagen with Runner's Drive	10 reps per side, 1–2 sets	258
Intermediate	Modified Copenhagen on Jump Box	1–2 sets per side	231

WEEK TWENTY–THREE: Hip Strength

This week we'll focus on building hip strength to support your changing posture and enhance pelvic stability.

Note: Keep your standing knee soft, avoid leaning sideways, and use fingertip support as needed for the following exercises, especially as pregnancy shifts your center of balance.

LEVEL	EXERCISE	SETS × REPS	PAGE
Beginner	Seated Hip Abduction	10 reps, 1-2 sets	236
Intermediate	Seated Hip Abduction (Banded)	10 reps, 1-2 sets	236
Beginner	Standing Hip Abduction	10 reps per side, 1-2 sets	252
Intermediate	Standing Hip Abduction (Banded)	10 reps per side, 1-2 sets	253

WELLNESS INSIGHT
Thank you notes are in your future! Consider purchasing some in advance for any upcoming baby showers and for after your baby arrives.

EQUIPMENT
• Chair
• Stable surface for support
• Loop band
• Long resistance band

FREQUENCY
3 days per week

WEEK TWENTY–FOUR: Hip Stability

This week you'll work on strengthening the muscles that stabilize your hips from multiple angles, ensuring a solid foundation for your body.

LEVEL	EXERCISE	SETS × REPS	PAGE
Beginner	Side-Lying Hip Abduction	10 reps per side, 1-2 sets	240
Intermediate	Side-Lying Hip Abduction (Banded)	10 reps per side, 1-2 sets	240
Advanced	Glute Wall Reach	10 reps each side, 1-2 sets	222

WELLNESS INSIGHT
Your baby will be here before you know it. Celebrate moments of calm, and prioritize time with loved ones.

EQUIPMENT
• Loop band
• Wall
• Mat

FREQUENCY
3 days per week

WEEK TWENTY-FIVE: Movement Control

EQUIPMENT
• Loop band

FREQUENCY
3 days per week

This week's exercises focus on controlled lateral movement patterns, which help enhance stability as your center of gravity continues to shift. These side step movements are particularly beneficial during pregnancy because they strengthen your pelvis and hip muscles as they adapt to carry your growing baby. Lateral movements also improve your balance and coordination, helping you feel more confident navigating daily activities like getting in and out of cars, moving around furniture, or simply changing direction while walking.

LEVEL	EXERCISE	SETS × REPS	PAGE
Beginner	Side Steps	10 reps each direction, 1-2 sets	244
Intermediate	Side Steps (Banded)	10 reps each direction, 1-2 sets	244

WEEK TWENTY-SIX: Glute Activation

WELLNESS INSIGHT
While you still have
weeks to go, now
is a good time to
start packing the
essentials for your
birth center bag.

EQUIPMENT
• Loop band
  (optional)
• Mat

FREQUENCY
3 days per week

In the final week of your second trimester, you'll focus on deep glute activation to support pelvic stability and ensure proper leg alignment during daily movements.

LEVEL	EXERCISE	SETS × REPS	PAGE
Beginner	Side-Lying Clamshells	10 reps per side, 1-2 sets	239
Intermediate	Side-Lying Clamshells (Banded)	10 reps per side, 1-2 sets	240
Advanced	Kneeling Side Plank Clamshells	10 reps per side, 1-2 sets	227

LOOKING AHEAD

As we wrap up the second trimester, take a moment to reflect on how far you've come. This phase of pregnancy has likely brought significant physical and emotional changes.

You've learned to modify your fitness routine by staying attuned to your needs as you master new exercises. By identifying people and professionals who can help guide you through this journey, you've strengthened your support system. And you've made time for self-reflection, prioritizing your mental and emotional well-being alongside your physical health.

Remember, the goal is progress, not perfection. Every small step you take—whether it's mastering a new pregnancy-safe exercise, having an important conversation with your healthcare provider, or simply taking time to connect with your growing baby—is a victory worth celebrating.

As you enter your third trimester, carry forward the habits and insights you've gained so far throughout your pregnancy journey. Stay active while always listening to your body and adjusting as needed, and continue nurturing your support system—you'll rely on them even more in the months ahead. Keep communicating openly with your healthcare team, sharing any concerns and questions that arise during this final phase. Take time for self-care and reflection, remembering that your mental health is just as important as your physical health. Most importantly, stay flexible and open-minded, knowing that it's okay if your journey doesn't unfold exactly as you imagined.

The third trimester will bring its own challenges and joy. You'll be preparing for birth, managing the physical demands of late pregnancy, and getting ready to meet your baby. But with the progress you've made during the second trimester, you're well-equipped to handle whatever comes your way.

PART IV

THE THIRD TRIMESTER

CHAPTER 10

Preparing for Birth and Beyond

Welcome to the third trimester! This is the final stretch of your pregnancy, which will bring new developments. As your baby rapidly gains weight, you'll feel the increasing effects of sharing your space. Many women joke that nature signals you're ready for birth by making you feel tired of sharing your body. While these discomforts can be challenging, try to embrace and savor these final weeks of pregnancy.

You may find that time moves at varying speeds—some moments will seem to crawl past as you eagerly await holding your baby, while others fly by, leaving you to wonder if you're truly prepared for your baby's arrival. Rest assured, it's completely natural to experience a wide range of emotions during this time. We're here to support you through it all.

YOUR BODY'S NEW NORMAL

Understanding third-trimester changes can help you work with your body rather than against it, allowing you to be as comfortable as possible while preparing for your baby's birth.

Breathing and Circulation

During this phase your respiratory system adapts to support both you and your baby. Your ribs may rise about two inches toward your collarbone, which can cause tingling or numbness in both hands, while your rib cage widens, affecting how your clothes fit around your torso. You may also feel out of breath more easily during daily activities, which is a common occurence as your body works harder to provide oxygen for two.

Your body adapts to these changes in remarkable ways. By exercising during your pregnancy, you're supporting these adaptations, which include:

- Improved oxygen uptake to meet the needs of your baby, placenta, uterus, and heart
- Enhanced carbon dioxide elimination
- Increased tidal and respiratory volume (the amount of air moving in and out of your lungs and their total capacity)
- A higher respiratory rate (the number of breaths you take per minute)
- A 40 to 50 percent increase in heat dissipation due to more frequent breathing

Temperature Regulation and Exercise

In the third trimester your body becomes highly efficient at regulating temperature. Heat dissipation improves as your body weight increases, providing more skin surface area, while enhanced blood vessel networks support cooling.

Exercise during pregnancy further boosts temperature regulation. You can maintain a safe core temperature by adjusting your exercise intensity, aiming for 65 percent of your maximum capacity. However, due to changes in blood volume during late pregnancy, reaching a higher heart rate can be more challenging in your third trimester. To monitor intensity during this time, consider using the Borg RPE scale to gauge perceived exertion instead of tracking your heart rate. You could also do the talk test or just incorporate adequate rest periods and check in with yourself.

Pelvic Floor Changes

As your baby grows, your pelvic floor continues its preparations for birth. Hormonal shifts increase flexibility, allowing the pelvic floor muscles to adapt more easily. At the same time, these muscles face increased demands due to postural changes and the weight of your growing abdomen.

Jessica's Pelvic Floor Insights

Understanding the balance between strength and relaxation is crucial at this stage. Focus on conscious relaxation exercises that help your pelvic floor release tension, gentle strengthening movements that maintain function without overworking these muscles, birth position practice to prepare your body for delivery, and perineal preparation techniques that support tissue flexibility during birth.

Weight Distribution and Posture

As your center of gravity continues changing, your body continues to adjust to maintain stability and balance. Your lumbar spine may curve more to accommodate your growing belly, while your hip joints become more mobile to support this shifting weight. Meanwhile, your lower back muscles work harder to provide stability, and your feet may change in both size and shape as they adapt to carrying additional weight and hormonal changes affecting your ligaments.

Sleep and Rest in the Third Trimester

Just when you feel you need it most, sleep often becomes more elusive. Your body is preparing you for life with a newborn, but this doesn't make third-trimester nighttime challenges any easier. Many women find themselves tossing and turning, struggling to find a comfortable position, only to need another bathroom visit as soon as they've settled.

While disturbed sleep is normal during this time, understanding its causes can help you develop effective strategies. The weight of your growing baby, combined with hormonal changes, anxieties, and excitement about impending motherhood, all contribute to sleep disruption. However, there are ways to improve the quality of your rest.

SLEEP SOLUTIONS

As a reminder, you can help yourself sleep better by:

- Establishing bedtime routines
- Practicing relaxation techniques
- Managing your fluid intake in the evening
- Creating a comfortable sleep environment

The key to better sleep lies in preparation. Transform your bedroom into a sleep sanctuary with proper temperature control and supportive pillows. A pregnancy pillow or a strategic pillow arrangement can help support your abdomen, joints, and ligaments. Try placing one pillow between your knees to align your hips, another under your belly for support, and one behind your back to prevent rolling.

Common Discomforts and Solutions

As pregnancy progresses, various discomforts can arise. Understanding why these discomforts occur can help you approach them with patience and find practical solutions. Maintaining good posture becomes increasingly important, although it will require conscious effort at this stage of your pregnancy.

Common third-trimester challenges include:

- Swelling in your feet and ankles
- Heartburn and indigestion
- Shortness of breath
- Hip and pelvic discomfort

The good news is that most of these discomforts can be managed effectively. For example, regular, gentle movement can help reduce swelling, while proper body mechanics may ease back strain. Additionally, eating small, frequent meals is often more effective for managing heartburn than having three larger ones. Braces, support splints, and manual therapy can also help address hip, pelvic, and back pain.

Preparing for Birth

In Chapter 13 we will go into detail about creating a birth preference plan. Before we dive into that, however, here are some important things to consider as you enter your third trimester.

Expanding Your Healthcare Team

Now is the time to expand your healthcare team to include support for your postpartum journey. Consider adding the following professionals and groups to your network:

- Lactation consultant
- Urogynecology consultant
- Pediatrician
- Postpartum or night support provider
- Day care, nanny, or babysitter
- Moms' support group, fitness group, or social group

LOOKING AHEAD

Creating Your Nest

The nesting instinct—that powerful urge to prepare your home for your baby's arrival—is a natural and beneficial part of pregnancy. While it can arise at any time, many women experience stronger nesting urges during the third trimester. This surge of productive energy can help you accomplish important tasks, but it's important to channel it wisely.

Two Weeks Before

- Add fresh items to your birth center bag.
- Confirm your support team's availability.
- Prepare and freeze meals.
- Review your birth preferences with your birth partner.

One Week Before

- Stock up on fresh groceries.
- Arrange for house cleaning assistance.
- Attend the final medical appointments.
- Have your birth ball and comfort items ready.
- Prep your camera or phone for capturing memories.
- Charge all your devices.

PREPARATION PRIORITIES FOR STRATEGIC NESTING

- Purchasing essential baby items
- Taking measures to ensure home safety
- Planning meals
- Organizing your support system

Balance productive periods with adequate rest. When you feel a burst of nesting energy, focus on one manageable project at a time, such as preparing the baby's sleep space or organizing baby clothes by size. While nesting is natural and helpful, it shouldn't override your body's need for rest. Pay attention to signs of fatigue—they're your body's way of saying it needs a break to continue supporting you and your baby effectively.

Rachel Schneider Smith

Olympian

My biggest concern about maintaining fitness during pregnancy was ensuring that my training wouldn't harm my baby. As a professional runner who represented the US at the 2019 World Championships and 2021 Tokyo Olympics, I was used to pushing my body to its limits. But pregnancy required a completely different approach—one that prioritized intuition over intensity.

I built a trusted team of healthcare professionals, including my ob-gyn and prenatal physical therapist Jessica, who understood me as both an individual and an elite athlete. I learned to truly listen to my body and trust what felt right.

I was surprised by how much my body could still enjoy training throughout pregnancy. In my first trimester, I backed off mileage due to fatigue but still managed 60-70 miles weekly. My second trimester brought better energy levels—some days I'd run four miles, others fourteen, depending on how I felt. By the third trimester, I focused on easy miles and occasional cross-training, stopping at 37 weeks.

I took each day as it came without being attached to any specific training plan. I did what felt good and right for that moment.

I intentionally refrained from setting comeback expectations in postpartum. Freed from stress, I experienced a surprisingly smooth return—walking within days of giving birth, biking within two weeks, and running on an anti-gravity treadmill by four weeks. At six weeks postpartum, I was running on the ground again while breastfeeding and adapting to disrupted sleep.

My advice to other athletes: listen to your body and consult healthcare professionals who understand you as an individual. Our bodies possess incredible wisdom. When we listen, they tell us when to back off and when to push.

Now, I have profound reverence for what the female body can accomplish. I'm in constant awe of my daughter and the fact that my body nurtured her into existence. Pregnancy and motherhood didn't diminish my athletic identity—they expanded my understanding of what true strength looks like.

CHAPTER 11

Your Third-Trimester Exercise Program

As your baby grows and your body prepares for birth, exercise becomes less about performance and more about ensuring purposeful movement that supports your changing needs.

Note: Remember to revisit the basic instructions for all exercise starting positions on pages 200-202. Maintaining proper form and technique is essential for an effective exercise program.

EXERCISE PRINCIPLES FOR LATE PREGNANCY

Listen to Your Body

- Your energy levels may vary significantly.
- Your sleep patterns may affect your exercise tolerance.
- Your need for rest may change from day to day.

Adjust Your Expectations

- Focus on quality over quantity.
- Modify your movements as needed.
- Celebrate what your body can do.

Fuel Your Movement

- Your body increasingly uses fat for energy and reserves sugar to nourish the baby, so eat easily digestible carbohydrates every 30–45 minutes during workouts to ensure adequate fueling.
- Stay well-hydrated.

Adjust Your Position

- Place a pillow behind your upper back to improve blood flow to your baby when performing exercises or activities on your back.

Note: Balance can become more challenging as your pregnancy progresses. Hold onto something during any exercises that feel unstable. When you return to these exercises postpartum, you can challenge your balance by gradually reducing or eliminating hand support.

WEEK TWENTY-SEVEN: Core Stability with Movement

Your new normal might look different in this final trimester. This week we'll focus on maintaining core connection while introducing controlled leg movements.

LEVEL	EXERCISE	SETS × REPS	PAGE
Beginner	Runner's Clamshells	10 reps per side, 1–2 sets	233
Intermediate	Runner's Clamshells (Banded)	10 reps per side, 1–2 sets	234
Advanced	Side Step Downs	10 reps per side, 1–2 sets	244

WELLNESS INSIGHT
Your exercise intensity may naturally decrease as you approach delivery. Honor these changes and respect your body's needs.

EQUIPMENT
• Wall
• Loop band (for banded variation)
• Low jump box (approximately 6 inches high)

FREQUENCY
3 days per week

WEEK TWENTY-EIGHT: Lower Body Strength

Maintaining strength in both the front and back of your thighs can help you propel forward. It also builds the leg strength you'll need for tasks like carrying your baby up and down stairs.

LEVEL	EXERCISE	SETS × REPS	PAGE
Intermediate	Seated Leg Extensions (Banded)	10 reps per side, 1–2 sets	237
Advanced	Front Step Downs	10 reps per side, 1–2 sets	221

WELLNESS INSIGHT
Consider washing your baby's clothes ahead of time so you're prepared for their first weeks at home.

EQUIPMENT
• Chair
• Loop band
• Low jump box (approximately 6 inches high)

FREQUENCY
3 days per week

WEEK TWENTY-NINE: Hip and Core Integration

WELLNESS INSIGHT
In late pregnancy your body uses more fat for energy, reserving sugar to nourish the baby. Be sure to eat carbohydrate-rich foods, like fruit or other easily digestible snacks.

EQUIPMENT
• Chair
• Loop band
• Weights (optional)

FREQUENCY
3 days per week

This week focuses on maintaining strength while practicing controlled movement patterns that support lifting your baby out of the crib and protecting your knees during postpartum activities.

Note: Weights are reintroduced this week. You can use kettlebells or free weights. Choose an appropriate weight that allows you to maintain good form throughout the allotted repetitions.

LEVEL	EXERCISE	SETS × REPS	PAGE
Intermediate	Seated Leg Curls (Banded)	10 reps per side, 1-2 sets	237
Advanced	Split-Stance Romanian Deadlifts	10 reps per side, 1-2 sets	251

WEEK THIRTY: Balance and Stability

EQUIPMENT
• Long resistance band
• Stable surface for support

FREQUENCY
3 days per week

As your center of gravity continues to shift, these exercises will help you stay confident when standing on unstable surfaces.

Note: For the following exercises, keep your standing knee slightly bent, avoid leaning sideways, and use fingertip support as needed, especially as pregnancy changes shift your center of balance.

LEVEL	EXERCISE	SETS × REPS	PAGE
Beginner	Four-Way Ankle (Banded)	10 reps in each direction per side, 1-2 sets	220
Beginner	Single-Leg Balance	30 seconds, 2 reps per side, 1-2 sets	245
Intermediate	Single-Leg Balance Clock Reaches	5 reps per side, 1-2 sets	245
Advanced	Runner's Balance Challenges	10 reps per side, 1-2 sets	232

WEEK THIRTY-ONE: Upper Body Strength

This week we'll focus on maintaining upper body strength with exercises that support good posture as your belly grows. These exercises will also help build shoulder blade strength, which will be beneficial for lifting and carrying your baby.

EQUIPMENT
• Long resistance band

FREQUENCY
3 days per week

LEVEL	EXERCISE	SETS × REPS	PAGE
Beginner	Rows (Banded)	10 reps, 1-2 sets	232
Intermediate	Split-Stance Row (Banded)	10 reps per side, 1-2 sets	252
Advanced	Single-Leg to Single-Arm Row (Banded)	10 reps per side, 1-2 sets	250

WEEK THIRTY-TWO: Arm Strength

This week you'll work on maintaining upper body strength while practicing core stability in standing positions, preparing you for hours of holding, carrying, and lifting your baby.

WELLNESS INSIGHT
Make sure your car seat is properly installed and ready to go. Many places offer inspections to ensure it's securely fitted.

EQUIPMENT
• Long resistance band
• Weights

FREQUENCY
3 days per week

LEVEL	EXERCISE	SETS × REPS	PAGE
Intermediate	Triceps (Banded)	10 reps, 1-2 sets	257
Advanced	Front Arm Raises (Weighted)	10 reps, 1-2 sets	220

WEEK THIRTY-THREE: Shoulder Stability

EQUIPMENT
• Long resistance
  band
• Weights
• Chair
• Wall

FREQUENCY
3 days per week

This week's exercises focus on maintaining upper body strength to support good posture while also challenging your core. Be sure to engage your entire core throughout each exercise to maintain proper form and control.

LEVEL	EXERCISE	SETS × REPS	PAGE
Beginner	Pull Downs (Banded)	10 reps, 1-2 sets	232
Beginner	Seated Shoulder Press (Weighted)	10 reps, 1-2 sets	239
Intermediate	Diagonal Pulls (Banded)	10 reps per side, 1-2 sets	216
Intermediate	Wall Push-Up Plus	10 reps, 1-2 sets	258

WEEK THIRTY-FOUR: Modified Core Work

WELLNESS INSIGHT
Talk to your healthcare provider about when to go to the hospital after contractions have started. Keep the hospital address handy and consider doing a practice run to familiarize your-self with the route before the big day.

EQUIPMENT
• Mat
• Long resistance
  band
• Padded surface
  for knees

FREQUENCY
3 days per week

As your belly continues to grow, we'll focus on strengthening the smaller stabilizing muscles that play an important role in activating your entire core.

LEVEL	EXERCISE	SETS × REPS	PAGE
Beginner	Four Point Arm Lifts	10 reps per side, 2 sets	219
Intermediate	Four Point Leg Lifts	10 reps per side, 2 sets	219
Intermediate	Four Point Opposite Arm and Leg Lifts	10 reps per side, 2 sets	219
Advanced	Kneeling Pallof Press (Banded)	10 reps per side, 1-2 sets	226

WEEK THIRTY-FIVE: Calf Relief

During these final weeks, we'll focus on relieving tightness in the calves, as your ever-growing belly places additional demands on these muscles to help keep you upright.

EQUIPMENT
• Wall

FREQUENCY
3 days per week

EXERCISE	SETS × REPS	PAGE
Calf Stretch	30 seconds per side, 1-2 sets	213
Bent-Knee Calf Stretch	30 seconds per side, 1-2 sets	211

WEEK THIRTY-SIX: Hip and Thigh Release

This week's stretches promote mobility and comfort in your hip muscles, helping them sustain the increased demands from your widening pelvis. They will also help prepare your body for labor positions.

Note: Balance may be more challenging in the third trimester. Be sure to have something to hold onto to ensure safety.

WELLNESS INSIGHT
You're likely getting tired on your feet, but sitting too much can position baby's head against your back (occiput posterior), which isn't ideal for descending through the birth canal. Change positions, take light walks, and stand up frequently.

EQUIPMENT
• Bench/stool/chair
• Stable surface for support

FREQUENCY
3 days per week

EXERCISE	SETS × REPS	PAGE
Dynamic Adductor Stretch	10-15 reps per movement, per side, 1-2 sets	217
Standing Hip Flexor Stretch	30 seconds per side, 1-2 sets	254
Standing Quadricep Stretch	30 seconds per side, 1-2 sets	255

WEEK THIRTY-SEVEN: Thoracic Mobility

WELLNESS INSIGHT
Women who exercise tend to have labors that are fifty minutes shorter and occur five to seven days earlier. As your due date approaches, rest whenever possible.

EQUIPMENT
• Chair
• Mat

FREQUENCY
3 days per week

This week we'll focus on exercises designed to help you maintain upper back mobility, which supports better posture and breathing.

EXERCISE	SETS × REPS	PAGE
Seated Twist Stretch	30 seconds per side, 1-2 sets	239
Side-Lying Rotation Stretch	30 seconds per side, 1-2 sets	241
Thread Needle Stretch	30 seconds per side, 1-2 sets	257

WEEK THIRTY-EIGHT: Birth Position Preparation

WELLNESS INSIGHT
Women retain six to eight liters of fluid during pregnancy, which gradually disappears within seven to ten days after delivery. Expect night sweats—keep a towel on your bed and extra pajamas nearby.

EQUIPMENT
• Mat
• Counter/table
• Foam roller

FREQUENCY
3 days per week

As your spinal curve continues to change—increasing strain on your back—this week's movements help maintain upper and lower back mobility. The first two exercises also mimic labor positions, helping you prepare for childbirth.

EXERCISE	SETS × REPS	PAGE
Child's Pose Stretch	30 seconds per position, 1-2 sets	214
Counter Stretch	30 seconds per position, 1-2 sets	215
Foam Roller Upper-Back Stretch	1-2 sets	218

WEEK THIRTY-NINE: Upper Body Release

This week, our focus is on maintaining shoulder and chest mobility. Your front chest muscles face increased strain—first from pregnancy-related postural changes and later from holding a baby for hours. Learning to open up these muscles can be a key exercise if you're feeling tension or tightness.

EXERCISE	SETS × REPS	PAGE
Standing Snow Angels	10 reps, 1-2 sets	256

WELLNESS INSIGHT
Remember that you will need to add your baby to your medical insurance soon.

EQUIPMENT
• Wall

FREQUENCY
3 days per week

WEEK FORTY: Birth Preparation

During this final week, we'll focus on reducing neck tension, which can intensify between contractions, and reminding you how to tilt your pelvis forward and back. These movements will help you gain more body awareness during labor and delivery.

EXERCISE	SETS × REPS	PAGE
Scalene Stretch	30 seconds per side, 1-2 sets	235
Seated Pelvic Tilts on Ball	10 reps, 2 sets	238

WELLNESS INSIGHT
As you approach (or pass) your due date, stay as active as you can while allowing yourself plenty of rest. Your body is doing important work in preparation for labor and delivery.

EQUIPMENT
• Therapy Ball

FREQUENCY
3 days per week

PART V

BIRTH PREPARATION AND EMPOWERMENT

CHAPTER 12

Understanding Labor and Delivery

Giving birth is an endurance event—one in which understanding each phase can help you work with your body rather than against it. Like elite athletes who tailor their approach specifically to each segment of a competition, knowing what to expect during every stage of labor allows you to adjust your strategy, conserve energy, and stay confident throughout your birth journey.

This deep understanding forms the foundation of an empowered birth experience. While every birth unfolds uniquely, recognizing the distinct characteristics and purposes of each phase helps you and your support team make informed decisions in the moment.

In the chapters ahead, we'll explore the complete labor and delivery journey, equipping you with a clear understanding of the four distinct stages of labor and their purposes, along with tools for recognizing the signs of progression. You'll gain evidence-based knowledge that empowers informed decision-making and a comprehensive overview of pain management options, from breathing techniques to medical interventions.

We'll provide practical guidance on common procedures and unexpected scenarios, specific techniques for optimal pelvic floor preparation, and effective pushing techniques that work with your body's natural processes. You'll also learn pelvic movements to facilitate labor and delivery, guidelines for active birth partner involvement, and strategic positions that assist labor progression. Finally, we'll cover effective communication strategies for working collaboratively with your healthcare team throughout this transformative experience.

This knowledge will help you build your birth toolkit—one that enables you to remain flexible while staying true to your preferences and needs. Whether your labor progresses quickly or slowly, whether you choose unmedicated or medicated pain management, understanding these fundamentals will empower you to navigate your unique path with confidence.

THE ATHLETIC MINDSET: LABOR'S NATURAL RHYTHM

Labor as Interval Training

Just as an athlete taps into the power of interval training, your body orchestrates labor through its own perfectly designed interval system. This natural pattern of work and recovery enables you to draw on incredible strength reserves and endurance that you might not even realize you have.

YOUR WORK INTERVALS: CONTRACTIONS

- Each contraction represents a focused effort and typically lasts 45 to 90 seconds.
- Like the segments in interval training, each contraction progressively increases in intensity.
- Your body should send clear signals when it's time to engage.
- Every contraction brings you closer to meeting your baby.

YOUR RECOVERY PHASES: BETWEEN CONTRACTIONS

- These crucial rest periods allow you to regroup and recharge.

- Although recovery phases shorten as labor progresses, these moments remain vital for restoring strength.
- Each rest phase offers opportunities for position changes, hydration, and a mental reset.

THE PROGRESSIVE CHALLENGE

- Early labor often feels like a warm-up, with gentler, more spaced-out contractions.
- Active labor brings more regular, powerful intervals.
- The transition phase represents your peak intensity.
- The pushing phase calls on your deepest resources.

YOUR EMPOWERED INTERVAL APPROACH

- Approach each contraction as a finite, manageable effort.
- Use recovery periods with purpose and intention.
- Have confidence in your body's natural pacing.
- Stay focused during intense moments.
- Find reassurance in the structured nature of the process.
- Be flexible if you need to pivot in unexpected circumstances.

While the birth process may be new to you, it is innate to your body. Each phase serves a specific purpose, and you can rely on your body's natural rhythm—and your knowledge—to support you through each interval.

THE FOUR STAGES OF BIRTH

Labor unfolds in four distinct stages, each with its own challenges. However, every stage also has a clear goal. Understanding these stages allows you to anticipate and work with your body's natural progression.

First Stage: Opening the Path

In this stage your body's primary focus is preparing the birth canal, progressing through three distinct phases. Each phase requires a different approach and energy management strategy.

EARLY LABOR PHASE

Think of early labor as your warm-up phase. During this phase your cervix gradually begins to open, and contractions start gently—sometimes weeks before delivery—often feeling similar to menstrual cramps. This is when you should rest and conserve energy for the work ahead.

ACTIVE LABOR PHASE

You'll find your rhythm as you move into active labor. Your cervix will continue dilating from 4 to 7 centimeters, typically over the course of 3 to 5 hours, although this timeline can extend for first births or with epidural use. Contractions become stronger and longer, lasting 45 to 60 seconds, but you'll have clear rest periods between them.

During active labor, movement becomes your ally. Changing positions every 30 minutes helps protect your body and encourages your baby's descent. This is also the ideal time to discuss pain management options with your healthcare team, including having an epidural if you're considering one, as these decisions become more challenging later in labor.

To maintain energy during this phase, focus on:

- Taking small sips of water between contractions
- Eating light, easily digestible snacks when possible
- Using rest periods to fully relax
- Communicating your needs clearly to your support team

TRANSITION: YOUR POWER PHASE

Transition is the intense final stretch of active labor before pushing. It's like the final sprint in a race, and it draws on your deepest strength reserves. This phase typically lasts between 30 minutes and 2 hours, during which you'll experience your most powerful contractions. These contractions often come one after another and last 60 to 90 seconds each.

Many women report feeling incredibly focused during transition, as if the rest of the world falls away. You might experience:

- Temperature fluctuations, shifting from hot to cold
- Nausea or vomiting
- Intense pressure in your back and pelvis
- Strong rectal pressure—an important signal to share with your team which may indicate that it's time for the pushing phase

If this is your second baby, transition may come sooner than expected.

The intensity of this phase serves a vital purpose: Your body is completing the final preparations for your baby's birth. Remember, you are strong, you are a mother, and your body has been preparing for this moment. In fact, your body will do much of the work for you. In the next steps in our journey together, you'll learn how to support your body in this phase by positioning your pelvis and relaxing your pelvic floor.

TRANSITION TOOLS

Prepare strategies for the following:

- Breathing through the intensity of your contractions
- Using support effectively
- Maintaining focus
- Working with your body
- Communicating your needs

THE STRATEGIC PAUSE: LABORING DOWN

After the intensity of transition, your body often takes a natural break—a phenomenon that might surprise you if you're not prepared for it. Once you reach full dilation at 10 centimeters, your contractions might briefly decrease in intensity. This isn't a sign that something is wrong; it's your body's wisdom at work, allowing both you and your baby a moment to prepare for delivery.

This laboring down phase can last anywhere from a few minutes to a couple of hours. Your healthcare team may encourage you to wait before pushing, allowing your baby to continue their descent naturally. This strategic pause often makes your pushing phase more effective when it begins. Trust your team's guidance during this time, as they're monitoring your baby's progress and will help you time your pushing efforts for optimal success.

Second Stage: Meeting Your Baby

The pushing phase brings your baby through the birth canal and into the world. This stage can last anywhere from minutes to several hours, and you'll work with your body's natural urges to push during contractions and rest between efforts. As your baby descends, you'll feel increasing pressure, culminating in the "ring of fire" sensation during crowning—the moment your baby's head becomes visible.

Like any endurance event, this stage has its own rhythm and progression. Pushing typically occurs during contractions, with rest periods between pushes allowing for recovery. Your team will provide guidance on timing and technique to help you through each phase of the process.

We'll explore specific pushing positions and techniques in more detail later, but for now, know that your healthcare team will guide you through this powerful phase. They'll prepare the delivery area and help you find effective positions for pushing.

Third Stage: Completing the Journey

Just as a race doesn't end when you cross the finish line—there's still the cool-down and recovery phase to consider—birth doesn't end the moment your baby is born. Those precious moments of holding your newborn for the first time may feel like the grand finale, but your body still has important work to do, starting with delivering the placenta. This remarkable organ, your baby's lifeline throughout pregnancy, has completed its job and is now ready to be released.

While this stage typically progresses smoothly, it requires careful attention. Postpartum hemorrhage (excessive bleeding) is rare but remains the leading cause of delivery-related complications, including maternal death. Your medical team will discuss two management approaches with you:

- **Active Management:** Using medical intervention to help deliver the placenta quickly and reduce the risk of bleeding
- **Passive Management:** Allowing your body to deliver the placenta naturally

In the moment, your healthcare provider will determine which approach best suits your situation. If needed, someone in your care team may massage your uterus to help it contract, and to prevent blood clots from forming. Be prepared—this can cause a strong, painful sensation.

Fourth Stage: Your Recovery Window

The first 24 hours after birth are paramount for healing and bonding. During this time you might experience:

- Physical shaking
- Continued uterine contractions
- Heightened awareness
- Increased adrenaline levels
- The powerful effects of skin-to-skin contact with your baby

Your medical team will monitor you closely, attending to any necessary perineal repairs and ensuring your stability.

FROM UNDERSTANDING TO PREPARATION

To prepare for the challenges of labor, it's important to focus on the natural changes your body will undergo and the intentional steps you can take to support the process. An athlete wouldn't attempt a marathon without training, and your delivery deserves the same level of attention. You've already built a strong foundation by understanding the four stages of labor. Now it's time to start preparing.

Preparing for Labor

Athletes reduce their training intensity before competition to recover and ensure they arrive at the starting line fresh and ready to compete. Similarly, your body will benefit from strategic preparation in the final weeks before birth. Focus on getting quality rest and sleep and ensuring you're eating plenty of nutritious foods. For exercise, reduce intensive activities and opt for gentle, consistent movement.

Starting around 20 to 30 weeks, and increasing in your last trimester, your body may go through its own practice sessions with Braxton Hicks contractions. These painless yet noticeable tightening sensations typically last 30 to 60 seconds and often increase with activity. Unlike true labor contractions, they usually ease when you change your position or increase your hydration levels.

MANAGING BRAXTON HICKS CONTRACTIONS

- Stay hydrated.
- Change positions.
- Take a warm bath.
- Practice relaxation techniques.
- Use them as opportunities to practice your birth preparation exercises.

Remember that Braxton Hicks contractions help your body prepare for labor. They're a normal and helpful part of pregnancy. However, if you're ever unsure whether you're experiencing Braxton Hicks or true labor contractions, contact your healthcare provider.

Knowing the difference between Braxton Hicks and true labor contractions helps you recognize when the real event begins. While Braxton Hicks contractions are irregular and often stop when you move or change your position, true labor contractions follow a predictable pattern and continue regardless of your activity. Braxton Hicks contractions are typically felt in the front of your abdomen, whereas true labor contractions may be felt in the low back, lower abdomen, and pelvis. Most notably, true labor contractions grow progressively stronger and closer together over time.

Recognizing Active Labor

While movies often dramatize a woman's water breaking as the signal that labor has begun, in reality, labor usually starts more subtly. Here are the main signals your body may give:

BOWEL CHANGES

When labor begins, your bowels might empty to prepare for delivery.

THE BLOODY SHOW

You may notice an increase in vaginal mucus, along with some blood in it, known as "the bloody show." This is a natural sign that labor is starting.

CONTRACTIONS

For most women contractions are faint and irregular to start with. As labor progresses, they become stronger, longer, and more frequent. Talk to your birth team to decide at what frequency and duration you should head to your birth center.

Here's how to time your contractions:

- Start timing from the beginning of one contraction to the start of the next.
- Note both the frequency and duration.
- Watch for increasing intensity.
- Track how long the pattern remains consistent.

Most medical teams recommend going to the hospital when contractions are 3 to 5 minutes apart, last 1 full minute, and have been consistent for 1 hour. For many first pregnancies, the 4-1-1 rule is a good guideline: head out when your contractions are 4 minutes apart, 1 minute long, and consistent for 1 hour—or if your water breaks!

If your water breaks, contact your birth team immediately to ensure you begin delivery early enough to prevent infection. Note the color, smell, and amount of fluid to help your medical team assess the situation. If you notice more blood than expected for the bloody show, or if you notice reduced fetal movement, go to the hospital right away.

EARLY LABOR FOCUS

During early labor, focus on:

- Relaxation techniques
- Proper hydration
- Energy conservation
- Quality nutrition
- Position changes

Arriving at Your Birth Center

When it's time to go to your birth center, call ahead to let them know you're on your way. This helps the staff prepare for your arrival and ensures you'll receive prompt attention. Once you arrive, you'll likely spend 20 to 30 minutes in triage while the medical team assesses you, determines if you are in active labor, and prepares your room.

Keep your birth center bag handy, as you might not go directly to your delivery room. Remember, this assessment time is a normal part of the admission process. Use it actively—you don't have to wait around.

Note: If you are not yet in active labor, the hospital might encourage you to go home or walk around nearby and provide guidance on when to return.

If you are admitted, don't feel like you have to sit still! Use the hospital environment to your advantage, as it offers many support options during early labor. Walking in the hallway keeps gravity working in your favor, and when contractions come, you can use handrails, countertops, or the backs of tall chairs to work through them. These stable surfaces provide excellent support for various labor positions.

LOOKING AHEAD: EXPLORING YOUR BIRTH PREFERENCES

Now that you understand the stages of labor, you can start developing your birth preferences. In the next chapter, we'll help you create a birth preference plan that honors your ideal vision while building in the flexibility needed for various scenarios.

You'll learn how to communicate effectively with your birth team, make informed decisions about common procedures, and prepare for unexpected situations while staying true to your preferences and remaining adaptable. We'll also guide you in working confidently with your support system throughout the entire process.

Think of this plan not as a rigid script but as a trusted guide—one that helps you navigate decisions with confidence while embracing labor's natural flow.

Jordan Hogan

Boston Marathon 2x bronze medalist

Strong as a Mother has been as essential to me in my pregnancy as a pair of running shoes is in a marathon buildup! As a first-time expectant mother, I had no idea what to do or where to begin when it came to staying fit and preparing my body for the incredible journey ahead. Now, as I near the birth of my baby, I feel completely prepared and confident—a feeling I never expected to have as a new mom.

Just as I would look back at my marathon training log to see how each workout built toward race day, I can look back at this book and everything I've done to prepare both my body and mind for birth. The systematic approach has given me the same confidence I feel toeing the start line of a big race, knowing I've done the work and trusted the process.

Throughout my first trimester, two exercises became absolutely essential to my daily routine. The core curl-ups taught me proper breathing technique and form, focusing on that crucial ribs-to-belly-button connection. I've made it a point to do at least one set daily, even before my runs, and I truly believe this foundation has allowed me to continue running all the way through my third trimester without discomfort. Equally important have been the pelvic floor foundational exercises, which I do religiously after my afternoon nap. I've experienced no pelvic floor discomfort while running, which I attribute entirely to this consistent work. More importantly, I know these exercises will be crucial for both birth and postpartum recovery.

As I moved into my second trimester, the ladder drills became a game-changer. Surprisingly, I actually felt like I was getting faster and my balance was improving during pregnancy—something I never thought would be possible! As my bump grew, these agility skills helped me navigate my changing body with confidence. The glute work also became increasingly important as my center of gravity shifted. Maintaining glute strength and balance has been key to preserving my power and stability as my body continues to change.

Now in my third trimester, I've shifted focus to upper body strength and stretching in preparation for carrying my little one. As my bump has expanded, my ribs have become sore, making the thoracic mobility work absolutely essential for comfort. I'm also beginning my birth preparation phase—starting perineal massage soon and finally cutting back on some of my heavier lifting. It feels exactly like marathon prep during taper time: trusting that I've done the work and now it's time to prepare for the big day.

The birth preference plan in particular makes me feel 100 percent confident for labor and delivery. I have nothing but excitement, determination, and a well-thought-out 'race plan' as I approach birth. Thank you so much, Jessica and Shannon, for sharing this invaluable resource with me and all mothers-to-be out there. I honestly don't know what I would do without this guidance—it's transformed my entire pregnancy experience from uncertainty to complete confidence.

CHAPTER 13

Your Birth Preference Plan

Understanding the stages of birth highlights an important truth: No matter how thoroughly you prepare, birth often unfolds unpredictably. That's why we use the term "preference" alongside "plan." This subtle shift in language encourages both confidence and flexibility during your birth journey.

Your birth preference plan should serve as a compass that guides you through your delivery, not a route set in stone. Preparation helps you make informed decisions, but adaptability is key to navigating the unpredictable process of birth. This balance between preparation and flexibility will become your greatest strength during labor.

Some mothers and their healthcare providers prepare detailed birth plans, while others prefer to have no plan at all. Both approaches have merit, but we recommend a middle ground: a framework that helps you understand your options, feel empowered to make informed choices, and stay flexible.

Ultimately, the way you approach birth is up to you. You can create your own plan, allow your birth team to make the decisions for you, choose to forego planning altogether, or settle somewhere in between.

CREATING YOUR FRAMEWORK

Your birth preference plan helps you prepare for the journey ahead and serves two essential purposes. First, it acts as a map that helps you outline your priorities and communicate them to your birth team. Second, your expanded knowledge serves as a compass, helping you navigate, so you can confidently adjust your path when needed. In the chapters ahead, we'll explore each component of this framework in detail, helping you express your preferences and make informed decisions during labor and delivery.

Understanding Your Core Priorities

Start by establishing your fundamental goals, such as:

- Ensuring a healthy outcome for you and your baby
- Being able to make informed decisions
- Having confidence in your support system
- Being able to adapt while staying centered

Using these goals as a foundation, consider your preferences regarding:

- Comfort and pain management approaches
- Movement and positioning strategies
- Roles and responsibilities within your support team
- Communication styles and needs
- Environmental factors that help you feel secure

The Power of Flexible Strength

Remember, your birth preferences are a framework, not a mandate. The key to a positive birth experience is your ability to adapt while staying true to your core priorities. This flexibility is especially important when labor intensifies.

To build this adaptability, focus on:

- Identifying your non-negotiables
- Exploring alternative or backup options
- Developing confidence in your support team

- Keeping communication channels open
- Taking confidence in your preparation

In the Birth Preference Plan, we'll look at tools and techniques that support this flexible framework—from optimal positioning to effective communication with your birth team. Each element builds on the last, creating a comprehensive strategy that honors your preferences and the natural flow of birth.

The Science Behind Mental Preparation

Thorough preparation can have a positive impact on both your body and mind during birth. Understanding the birth process helps activate the rational part of your brain, reducing the fight-or-flight response. This mental readiness triggers a cascade of positive physical effects.

Your Body's Hormonal Dance

There are two hormones that play vital roles during delivery.

OXYTOCIN: YOUR NATURAL ALLY

Often referred to as the love hormone, oxytocin supports:

- Labor progression
- Effective contractions
- Natural pain management
- Mother–baby bonding
- Early milk production

CORTISOL: THE STRESS RESPONSE

While some stress is normal, excessive cortisol can:

- Make you feel tense, fearful, and protective
- Lengthen labor duration
- Affect your baby's heart rate
- Reduce the effects of natural pain management
- Impair decision-making abilities
- Decrease contractions
- Reduce blood flow to the uterus and placenta

Embracing Your Agency

Viewing birth as an active experience, rather than something that simply happens to you, changes how you approach decisions. Your agency exists on a spectrum—it's more than just consenting to or declining treatment. It also includes deciding how much information you wish to receive about every aspect of birth. You may choose to be deeply involved in some areas while delegating others to your healthcare team during critical decision-making moments.

This flexible approach empowers you to direct energy where it matters most, adapt to varying circumstances, be confident in your choices, collaborate effectively with your birth team, and preserve mental stamina throughout the entire experience.

Building Your Birth Vision

Take a layered approach to your birth preferences, with each layer supporting your ultimate goal of a healthy outcome. Below is an overview of the different layers.

FOUNDATION LAYER: CORE WELL-BEING

- You and your baby's physical health
- Your emotional well-being
- Basic safety needs

COMFORT LAYER: PERSONAL EXPERIENCE

- Pain management preferences
- Movement options
- Position choices

ENVIRONMENT LAYER: BIRTH ATMOSPHERE

- Support team composition
- Room ambience
- Communication preferences
- Documentation choices, such as taking photos or videos

Remember that your preferences represent flexible guidelines. Your healthcare team will work with you to ensure that your preferences support the safest and most positive birth experience possible.

PREPARING FOR INFORMED DECISIONS

Before creating specific preferences, it's important to understand your own situation and the options that are available to you. This knowledge will help you engage in meaningful discussions with your healthcare team. Let's explore some key considerations for an informed birth journey.

Assessing Your Individual Needs and Concerns

Start by reflecting on your particular circumstances and medical history, as these factors will inform your birth preferences and preparation strategies. Important medical considerations include previous injuries or surgeries, existing medical conditions, family health history, and any previous pregnancy experiences. You should also consider previous pelvic floor lacerations or episiotomies (surgical incisions made to assist with delivery), age-related factors, and any emotional or physical trauma that might influence your birth experience.

Common concerns surrounding birth often include pain management during labor and delivery, the risk of tearing during vaginal delivery, and the possibility of cesarean delivery or instrument-assisted delivery. Many women also have questions about vaginal birth after cesarean (VBAC) considerations and potential postpartum issues like urinary or bowel incontinence and prolapse. Understanding these possibilities ahead of time helps you prepare mentally and discuss options with your healthcare team.

Share your thoughts and concerns with your healthcare team early, as this enables them to help develop strategies tailored to your needs and to coordinate with specialists if necessary. If you have specific physical considerations, consulting a pelvic health specialist with obstetric experience can be invaluable. They can help you understand your specific needs, suggest position modifications, create targeted support strategies, and collaborate with your birth team to ensure you have a well-thought-out plan.

Pain Management: Understanding Your Options

Your views on pain management during birth are likely shaped by personal values, research, and conversations with others. While it's natural to feel drawn to a particular approach—such as an unmedicated birth or an epidural—keeping an open mind about all available options better prepares you for the unpredictable nature of labor and delivery. By understanding your pain management options, you can make informed decisions that prioritize your well-being during birth, even if circumstances require you to reconsider your initial preferences.

MYTH: Unmedicated birth is superior to medicated birth

Many women feel drawn to the idea of experiencing birth without an epidural or other pain management medications. This preference has shifted over time, shaped by changing cultural attitudes and evolving medical practices around labor and pain management. However, it's important to recognize that some women may measure the success of their birth experience primarily by whether they avoided pain medication, turning this personal medical choice into an achievement marker. While this perspective is understandable, it can create unnecessary pressure and overshadow the many other meaningful aspects of bringing your baby into the world.

THE TRUTH ABOUT EPIDURALS

Instead of viewing pain management as a binary choice between medicated or unmedicated birth, consider it a spectrum of tools that are available to support you during your delivery—each with its own benefits and considerations.

Current research highlights several benefits having an epidural: it can provide much-needed rest during long labors, may help manage anxiety for both you and your birth partner, may reduce the risk of pelvic floor tearing, and help conserve energy for the demanding work of labor and delivery.

Note: Epidurals usually don't limit you to lying on your back. You should still be able to choose side-lying, supported hands-and-knees, or birth-ball positions.

It's also important to consider these potentially undesirable effects of choosing to use an epidural: your labor may take longer, you'll need a catheter until the epidural wears off, and you may experience different sensations while pushing. Additionally, you'll need to change positions regularly, and your birth partner may need to help monitor the time spent in each position to ensure protection of your body throughout the process.

Note: There are medical risks involved with having an epidural. Be sure to discuss these with your healthcare team.

Alternative Options

NITROUS OXIDE

Nitrous oxide, often referred to as laughing gas, can offer a gentler, more temporary approach to medicated pain management. It helps reduce anxiety, doesn't impact mobility, acts quickly, and has minimal lasting effects, making it an appealing option for mothers who want some pain relief while maintaining control and movement during labor.

HYDROTHERAPY

Hydrotherapy offers an unmedicated option for pain management during labor. Whether you're in the shower or a birth tub, warm water provides natural relief and helps ease discomfort, promoting relaxation. You'll have the freedom to move and try different positions, which can enhance your sense of control. Hydrotherapy also encourages active involvement from your birth partner, and some facilities offer specialized birth tubs.

Rather than committing firmly to any single approach, consider becoming an informed decision-maker. By understanding all your options—both unmedicated and medicated—you empower yourself to collaborate with your birth team and make choices that best serve you and your baby in the moment. Remember, there's no reward for refusing support that could benefit you both.

Understanding Potential Medical Interventions

While birth often progresses naturally, being informed about possible interventions allows you to participate confidently in decision-making when needed.

KEY TIMING GUIDELINES

Your care team uses the following information, along with other factors, to guide recommendations during birth:

- Active pushing typically shouldn't exceed 95 minutes.

- Pelvic floor-related health risks increase by 23 percent for every 30 minutes beyond the initial 95 minutes.

FACTORS THAT MAY INFLUENCE CARE

Several factors might impact the need for medical intervention, including a history of pelvic floor lacerations, pre-existing injuries such as hip labral tears, hip impingement, neck and wrist issues, or disc herniations, the baby's position and size, and any medical complications that arise during labor.

ASSISTED DELIVERY

Sometimes your healthcare team might recommend assisted delivery as the safest approach for your baby's final descent. Use the following information to help you make informed decisions:

- **Vacuum Assistance:** Vacuum assistance generally carries a lower risk to your pelvic floor than forceps assistance.
- **Forceps:** In certain cases, forceps may be necessary to help expedite the delivery.

If your baby's head is large, delivery might be more difficult, which can increase the risk to your pelvic floor. In this case, your baby's size might be a bigger concern than the assistance method used.

Care providers will use different tools for different situations. Your healthcare team will explain why a particular method is recommended for your delivery.

Remember that labor can be unpredictable. Your healthcare provider can only inform you of risks that are known at the time of the decision.

Moving Forward with Confidence

Now that you understand your options and personal preferences, you've laid the groundwork for the journey ahead. Instead of viewing delivery as a test to pass or a performance to perfect, think of it as a profound experience that will unfold in its own unique way. Your role isn't to control everything but to make informed choices that support both you and your baby's well-being.

Take some time to reflect on what matters most to you about this experience. Perhaps it's feeling heard and respected throughout the process, maintaining a sense of calm despite the intensity, or ensuring your birth partner feels confident in their supportive role. While a healthy outcome remains paramount, acknowledging these additional hopes and preferences can help shape a more meaningful experience.

Consider exploring these thoughts in more detail using your pregnancy journal. Write about your ideal birth experience, and reflect on how you might respond if circumstances require a different approach. This reflection isn't about creating rigid expectations; it's about understanding your own priorities and building flexibility into your approach.

In the following chapters, we'll continue to help you deepen your knowledge and self-awareness. You'll learn how your birth partner can support you effectively by mastering positions that work with your body and facilitate labor and delivery. Most importantly, you'll develop the confidence to communicate your needs clearly while remaining open to the adaptability that birth requires.

Remember, your birth experience belongs to you and your baby. Whether you opt for a detailed birth preference plan or adopt a more fluid approach, success lies in feeling informed, supported, and empowered, every step of the way. There's no right way to give birth—only the way that best serves you and your baby in each moment.

BIRTH VISION QUESTIONS

Consider:

- What aspects of birth matter most to you?
- Which outcomes (beyond the foundation layer of health) feel important?
- What specific concerns need addressing?
- How will you balance your preferences with a flexible approach?

After delivery, it can be helpful to reflect on your answers to these questions to see how your expectations matched your experience.

CHAPTER 14

Essential Birthing Techniques

Your birth journey becomes more manageable when you master these five fundamental techniques:

- Pelvic floor relaxation
- Deep, low sounds
- Pelvic tilting
- Supportive pelvic pressure techniques
- Strategic positioning

By practicing these techniques before birth, you'll build confidence and capability. In the following chapters, we'll explore each one in detail.

RELAXING YOUR PELVIC FLOOR

Perhaps the most remarkable physical feat during delivery is your pelvic floor's ability to stretch up to 300 percent of its normal length. This incredible adaptation doesn't happen by chance; your body prepares for it through hormonal changes, and there are specific techniques you can use to support this process.

Perineal Stretching

To support your body's naturally increased pelvic floor flexibility, you can begin gentle perineal stretching once you reach thirty-four weeks of pregnancy (and after receiving clearance from your healthcare team). This technique helps prepare the *perineum* for birth and is particularly beneficial for first-time mothers.

Note: Your perineum is the space between your vagina and anus.

Before practicing, make sure your nails are clean and trimmed and that you've washed your hands thoroughly. Then, find a quiet, relaxed environment and a comfortable position, like lying in bed or sitting with one foot elevated.

BASIC TECHNIQUE

- Apply a water-based lubricant to your fingers, thumbs, and perineal area.
- Insert your thumb into your vagina, about 1 inch deep.

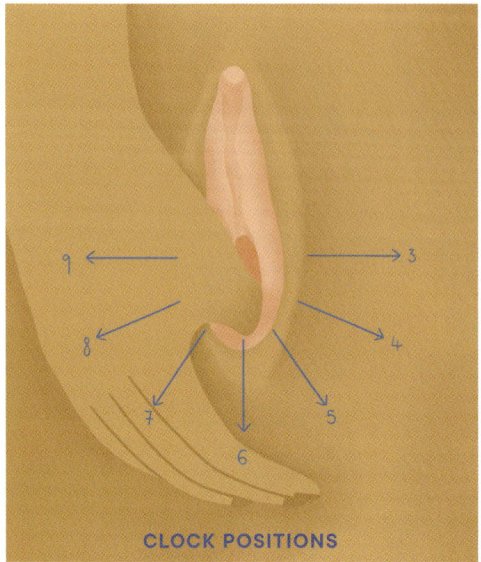

CLOCK POSITIONS

Practice these labor-supporting sounds, paying attention to which feel the most natural to you and how your body responds:

- Deep bear growl (GRRR)
- Low cow moo (MOOO)
- Calming om (OMMM)
- Gentle puppy pant (HAAA)
- Soothing shush (SHHH)

Your birth partner can help you relax by matching your pitch during a contraction and gradually lowering their tone, encouraging you to follow their lead.

- Apply gentle but firm downward pressure (toward your anus, repeating at clock positions 5 and 7) until you feel a stretch or slight burning sensation.
- Move your thumb down and side to side, massaging the bottom half of your vagina.
- Increase the pressure gradually, if comfortable.
- Practice this technique 3 to 5 times a week for 3 to 5 minutes.

ACTIVATING LOW-PITCHED SOUNDS

Your voice is a powerful tool during labor. Low, deep sounds help promote relaxation in your pelvic floor and body, while higher-pitched tones can increase tension.

HOW TO PUSH PROPERLY

To push effectively during labor, follow a sequence that works with your body's natural mechanisms. Begin with your breath, allowing your belly to expand fully while maintaining relaxed, steady breathing. This creates the foundation for effective pushing.

Next, focus on creating an opening by consciously relaxing your anus. Keep your pelvic floor in a lengthened position rather than contracting it. Use the low-pitched vocalization you've practiced to help maintain this openness. Remember to keep your throat and jaw relaxed, as tension in these areas can create tension throughout your pelvic region.

Once you've established this open, relaxed state, you'll add power to your push. Your pushes need to be strong enough to overcome the resistance of the pelvic floor muscles but not so strong that you contract them.

Gently draw your ribs downward while pulling your navel toward your spine to engage your entire core. Imagine working in harmony with your contractions rather than fighting their rhythm. Visualize your baby moving downward through the birth canal with each push. During labor, if your health-care team suggests increasing your effort, push with more directed force and intent.

You can enhance your core engage-ment using additional techniques. If birth bars are available, create gentle pulling pressure to give your muscles more leverage. In a hands-and-knees position, press your hands firmly into the bed and draw them slightly toward your feet—similar to the bear plank exercise you've practiced—to activate your core muscles more effectively.

Note: These steps naturally activate your entire core system, including the rectus abdominis, and help to direct more power to your pushes while main-taining proper form.

The Essential Rest Phase

As you've learned, relaxation is your secret weapon. During labor it helps produce oxytocin, the hormone that powers your contractions and promotes

bonding with your baby. It also triggers the release of endorphins, your body's natural pain relievers.

Between contractions, focus completely on recharging by:

- Scanning for areas of held tension (jaw, shoulders, hands, pelvic floor)
- Releasing all unnecessary tension
- Staying hydrated with small sips of water

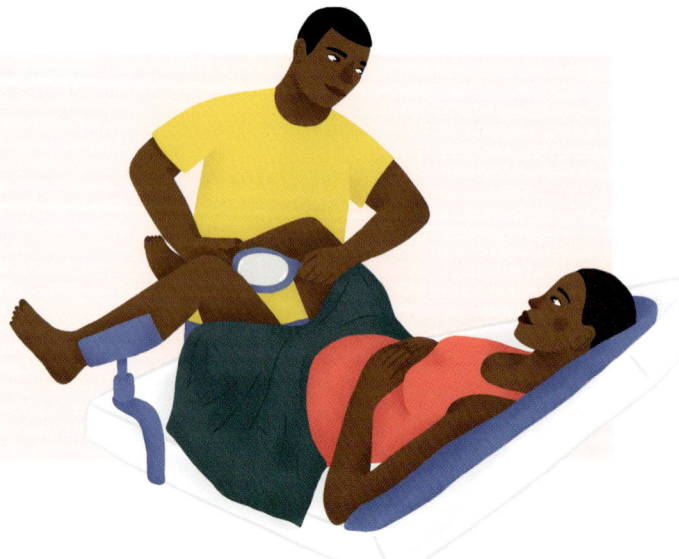

SEEING IS BELIEVING

Using a mirror can help you:

- Observe pelvic floor movement
- Notice the perineum lengthening
- Understand proper technique
- Build body awareness
- See your progress as the baby begins to crown

- Replenishing your energy with light snacks
- Being in the moment
- After each contraction, let go completely and treat each contraction as its own event. Your support team can help you track your rest phases to ensure you capitalize on their restorative potential.

FROM THE PRO
Shannon's Top Mental Tool for Birth—Relaxation

Just as I had a pre-race routine to get in the zone, I created a specific relaxation protocol for labor. Having these tools ready gave me confidence and helped me stay focused when things got intense.

We each have our own ways of staying motivated during challenging experiences. Athletes often use visualization to achieve peak performance, think through potential scenarios, or harness their emotions. You can use mental imagery to support your birth journey. Some women find it helpful to focus on things outside their bodies, while others prefer focusing inward.

HOW TO FOCUS OUTWARD

- Visualize running a familiar track, with each contraction representing an interval in a workout
- Think of each contraction as a wave carrying you closer to shore, where your baby waits to meet you.
- Consider each contraction a note in a symphony building toward the crescendo of your baby's arrival.

- Picture your baby's descent.
- Feel your pelvis opening.
- Picture your pelvic floor muscles relaxing.
- Focus on your breath.
- Notice your muscles relaxing.

Prepare for labor by experimenting with both internal and external visualization techniques during your pregnancy. Incorporate these mental exercises while holding challenging positions, during prenatal stretching, and throughout your regular work-out routines to build familiarity and effectiveness. You can also work collaboratively with your support team to refine these techniques, noting which approaches resonate most strongly with you.

In your pregnancy journal, keep a record of your most effective visualizations, preferred encouraging phrases, helpful metaphors, and ways your birth partner can help you maintain focus during labor. This preparation creates powerful mental tools you can call upon during the birthing process.

YOUR BIRTH ENVIRONMENT

Create a relaxing atmosphere by incorporating:

- Your favorite music playlist
- Calming scents
- Comfort objects
- Support from your birth team
- Familiar photos or focal points

Remember that what works during practice may change with the realities of labor. Stay flexible and open to trying different approaches as needed. In the next chapter, we'll explore specific positions to pair with these techniques throughout each phase of labor.

CHAPTER 15

Position and Movement During Birth

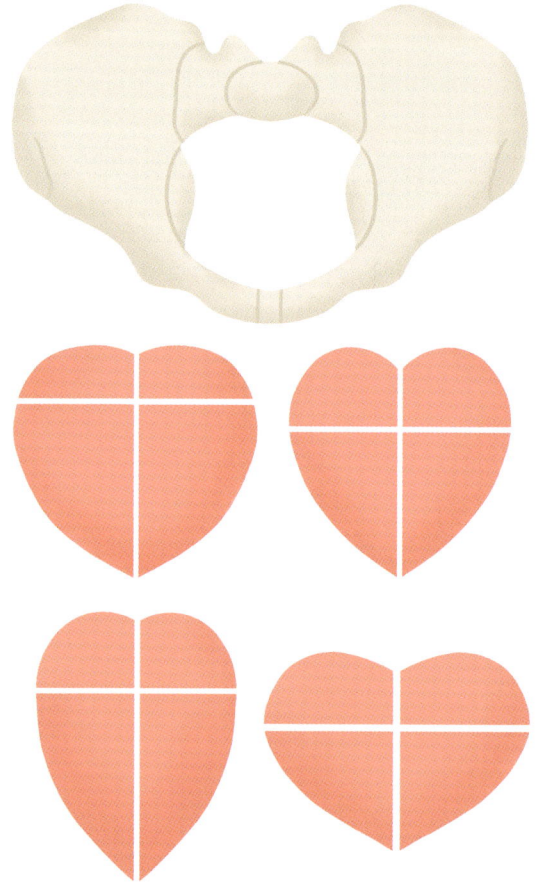

Your position during labor can dramatically influence your birth experience. By working with gravity and understanding how to move your pelvis, you can help ease your baby's journey.

THE SHAPE OF YOUR PELVIS

During childbirth, the baby navigates two key areas of the pelvis: the inlet and the outlet. The **pelvic inlet**, a ring of bones at the top of the pelvis formed by the pubis and sacrum, guides the baby during early labor. Later, during delivery, the baby passes through the **pelvic outlet**, formed by the tailbone and pubis.

Every person's pelvis has its own unique architecture. Some are more spacious from front to back, while others have a heart-shaped opening. These natural variations mean that finding effective positions may require some experimentation during labor. Depending on your pelvis shape, learning how to open your pelvis more front to back or more side to side may help facilitate your delivery.

WORKING WITH YOUR PELVIS

Regardless of your pelvic shape, certain movements and positions can help guide your baby downward.

To help the pelvic inlet open during labor contractions:

- Tuck your tailbone under you.
- Lean forward slightly.
- Create a gentle rounding in your lower back.

To help the pelvis outlet open during pushing contractions:

- Lift your tailbone.
- Arch your lower back slightly.
- Allow your pelvis to open.

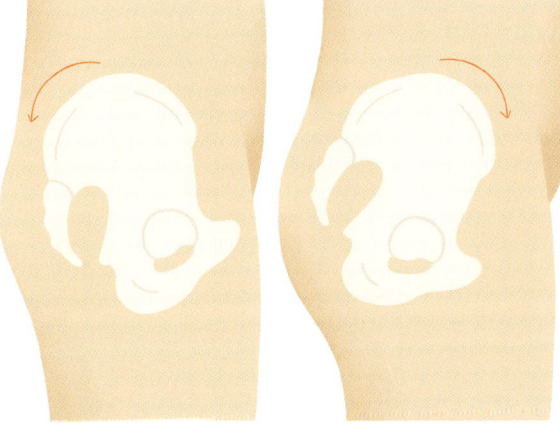

LABOR   DELIVERY

Gently keep your body active between contractions by:

- Moving your hips from side to side
- Rocking back and forth
- Staying in an upright position when possible

BIRTH PARTNER SUPPORT DURING LABOR AND DELIVERY

Communication

Before labor begins, establish clear signals with your birth partner and healthcare team to ensure smooth communication as the intensity builds. Consider creating:

- A specific word or gesture to signal when you want to discuss pain management options
- A clear signal for when you need to change positions
- A code word to inform your birth partner or doula when you're uncomfortable with staff interactions
- Boundaries for managing the outside world (social media updates, family communication, etc.)

These preparations help your birth partner advocate for you, request different staff members if needed, and manage family expectations and updates—allowing you to stay focused on giving birth.

Touch

Touch during labor serves multiple purposes. It stimulates helpful hormones such as oxytocin, provides comfort, and makes your uterine contractions stronger and more effective. Your birth partner can offer various levels of support, which we'll discuss on the following pages.

Early Labor Support

Let's take a look at two key techniques that your birth partner can use to support your baby's descent through the pelvic inlet.

SIDE-TO-SIDE PELVIC INLET SUPPORT

Have your birth partner:

- Place their hands on the greater trochanters (the small bumps on the sides of your hips)
- Squeeze gently, applying pressure toward the center of your pelvis to help create space for the baby's descent

FORWARD-BACK PELVIC INLET SUPPORT

Have your birth partner:

- Place one palm at the bottom of your sacrum (just above the fold of your gluteals) with their fingers pointing downward
- Position their other hand on the front of your pelvis
- Provide steady pressure to help the pelvic inlet open

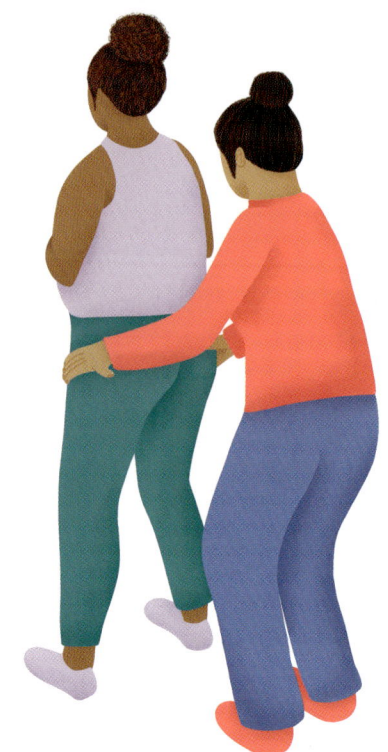

SIDE-TO-SIDE PELVIC INLET SUPPORT

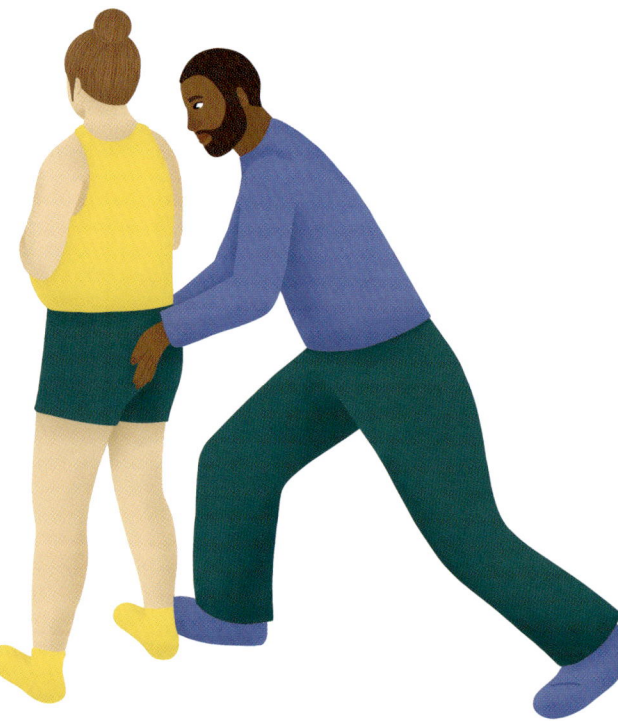

FORWARD-BACK PELVIC INLET SUPPORT

Pushing Phase Support

As birth approaches, your birth partner should adjust their support to help guide the baby's descent through the pelvic outlet.

SIDE-TO-SIDE PELVIC OUTLET SUPPORT

Have your birth partner:

- Move their hands just below the iliac crests (the curved ridges on the upper part of your hips)
- Apply gentle, steady pressure toward the center of your pelvis

FORWARD-BACK PELVIC OUTLET SUPPORT

Have your birth partner:

- Locate the sacral dimples just above your buttocks
- Place the heel of their hand below the dimples with their fingers pointing up
- Stabilize your pelvis by placing their other hand on the front of your hip
- Alter pressure (more or less) to match your needs as they change

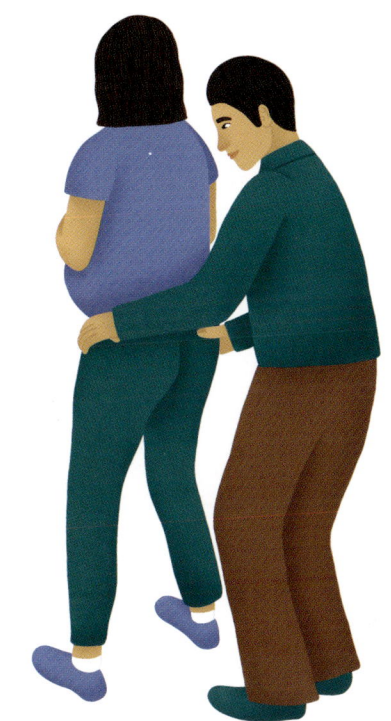

SIDE-TO-SIDE PELVIC OUTLET SUPPORT

PRACTICING BEFORE LABOR

Together with your birth partner, prepare for labor by:

- Learning the key pelvic pressure techniques
- Practicing different pressure intensities
- Noting which techniques feel most helpful
- Practicing smooth transitions

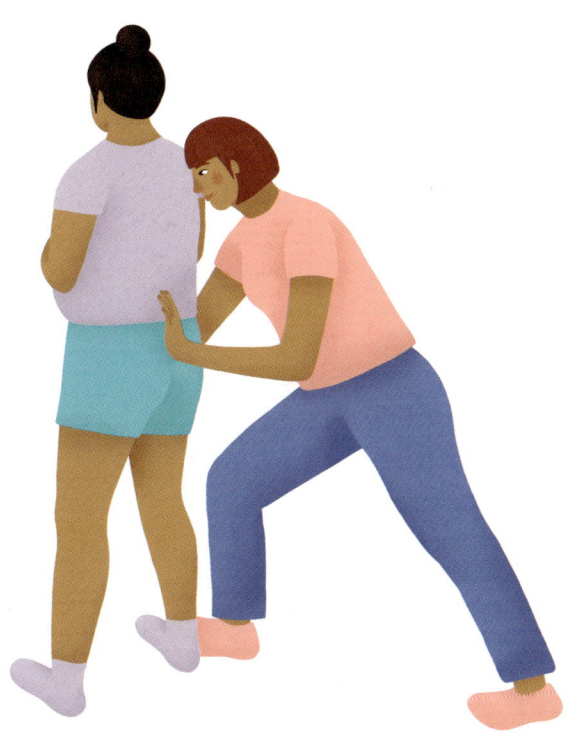

FORWARD-BACK PELVIC OUTLET SUPPORT

Comfort

Simple comfort measures your birth partner can provide include:

- Giving a gentle massage
- Stroking your hair
- Helping you release shoulder tension
- Holding your hand
- Encouraging you to relax your facial muscles
- Placing a hand on tense areas

POSITIONS FOR LABOR: A PROGRESSIVE JOURNEY

As your labor progresses, your positioning needs will naturally evolve. Think of these positions as tools in your birthing toolkit—each designed to serve a specific purpose and offer unique benefits. Instead of memorizing a long list of positions, focus on understanding the principles behind each type and how they can support you along the way.

Early Labor: Finding Your Rhythm

During early labor, movement is your greatest ally. Walking, swaying, and frequently changing positions can help your baby find their optimal path while keeping you comfortable. Try incorporating the time-tested approaches below during this phase.

DANCING WITH YOUR BIRTH PARTNER

One of the most intimate and effective positions for early labor involves working closely with your birth partner. Stand facing your birth partner, resting your hands on their shoulders or around their neck. Due to its intimate connection, this position provides both physical and emotional support. As your contractions intensify, lean into your birth partner and allow them to support your weight while you tuck your tailbone under and round your lower back. Between contractions, gentle swaying keeps you moving while helping to conserve energy.

THE SUPPORTED LEAN

Find a stable surface, such as a kitchen counter, the back of a couch, or a hospital bed raised to standing height. Lean forward, letting your arms and head rest while keeping your legs active. This position offers several benefits: it leverages gravity to aid your baby's descent, allows your partner to apply pelvic pressure techniques, and helps you fully relax between contractions. Many women naturally gravitate to this position, as it combines support with the instinctive urge to lean forward during contractions.

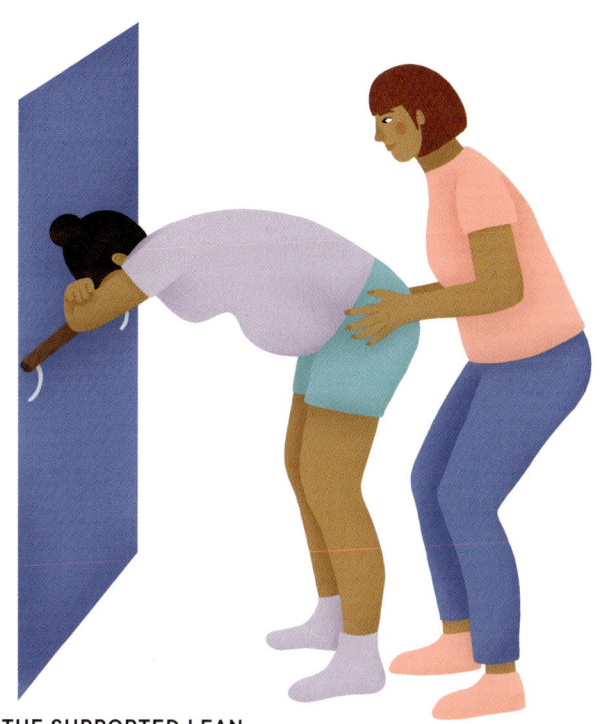

THE SUPPORTED LEAN

REFINING YOUR BIRTH POSITIONS

Start by learning the basic positions for labor. Once you feel confident, you can refine your technique by:

- Exploring the forward and backward tilt of your pelvis
- Consciously relaxing your pelvic floor
- Experimenting with different sounds
- Having your birth partner practice applying pelvic pressure techniques for labor and delivery in each position

Active Labor: Working with Intensity

As your labor intensifies, you may find yourself drawn to positions that provide more support while still harnessing the power of gravity. This is where various kneeling and seated positions become especially beneficial.

THE BIRTH BALL ADVANTAGE

A birth ball (large exercise ball) offers versatile support during active labor. You can:

- Sit and rock gently, allowing your pelvis to move freely
- Lean forward over the ball from a kneeling position to take pressure off your back

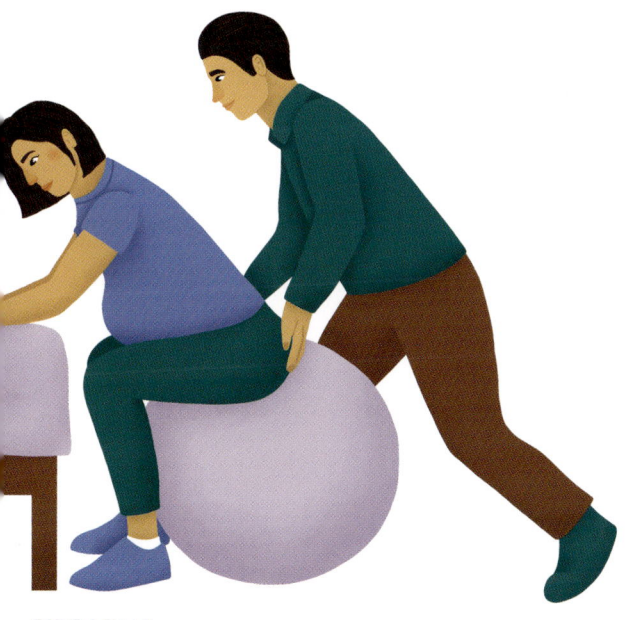

BIRTH BALL

- Use the ball for support while standing or kneeling to stay upright while conserving energy
- Your birth partner can provide steady pressure to your sacrum and hips while you use the birth ball, combining the benefits of positioning and touch support.

THE TOILET THRONE

While it might seem unconventional, sitting on a toilet (or birth ball) offers remarkable benefits during labor. This position naturally opens your pelvis while allowing you to face your birth partner for encouragement and stability. The familiar position also helps many people relax their pelvic floor—a key factor in labor progress. Your birth partner can provide extra support by applying gentle pressure to the front of your knees, which helps relieve pressure on your sacroiliac joints and the *pubic symphysis* (the joint where the two halves of the pubis come together).

HANDS AND KNEES: A GAME-CHANGING POSITION

Getting on your hands and knees is one of the most versatile and beneficial positions during labor. This position offers remarkable benefits, as it:

- Allows gravity to assist
- Provides pressure relief for sacroiliac and pubic pain

- Helps prevent tearing and protects previous perineal scars during delivery
- Allows excellent access for your birth partner to apply pelvic and hip pressure support
- Works with or without an epidural
- Can be used in both the labor and delivery phases

If your arms tire in this position, modify it by lowering yourself onto your forearms or resting your upper body on pillows or the raised head of the bed, tall-kneeling. From here, you can:

- Sway your hips side to side
- Rock back and forth
- Tuck your pelvis under for labor and arch your lower back during delivery
- Rest comfortably between contractions

Squatting is an instinctive laboring position for some. It opens your pelvis to its maximum capacity while utilizing gravity effectively. However, squatting during labor requires support—this isn't the time for independent squats. Your support options include:

- Holding onto your birth partner while they brace you from behind
- Using birth bars that are attached to the hospital bed
- Squatting against a wall, using pillows for comfort

- Using a specialized birth stool if your facility offers one
- The key is finding the right balance between opening your pelvis and your flexibility. Your team can help you modify this position to serve your needs.

Epidural Positioning

Having an epidural doesn't mean becoming passive during delivery. While movement may be more limited, you can still use positioning to your advantage by:

- Alternating sides every 30 minutes to prevent pressure points or nerve compression, as you won't feel these sensations
- Getting on your hands and knees (with assistance)
- Working with your team to find semi-upright positions for pushing

Remember to:

- Watch the contraction monitor to stay connected to your rhythm
- Use a mirror if you want to see your progress
- Have your support team assist with regular position changes
- Communicate any discomfort

The Power of Water During Labor

Whether you're using a shower or birth tub, water offers benefits during labor. Buoyancy and warmth can significantly affect your comfort level and mobility.

BIRTH TUB POSITIONING

If your facility offers a birth tub, consider these positions:

- Kneeling while leaning forward over the tub's edge
- Getting on your hands and knees with your belly submerged
- Sitting semi-reclined while being supported by your partner

Your birth partner can join you (wearing appropriate attire) to provide hands-on support, allowing you to combine the benefits of water, gravity, and touch.

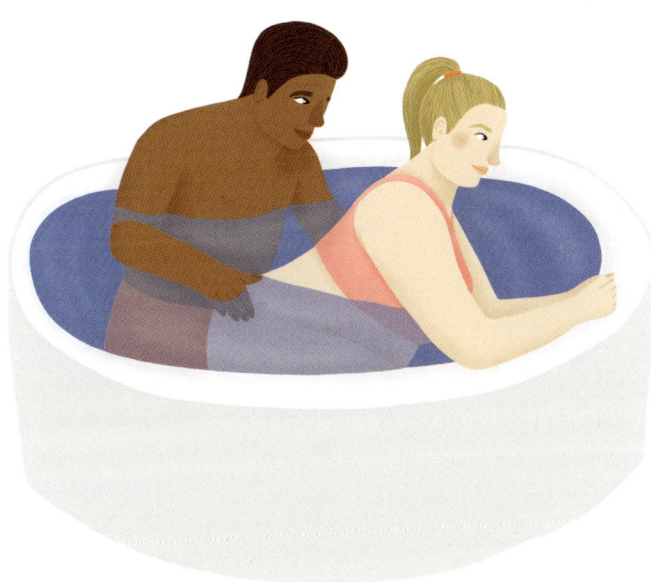

SHOWER POWER

Don't underestimate the humble shower as a labor tool. Many people find the shower more accessible and realize the better gravity benefits of the shower. You can:

- Stand and lean against the wall, letting the water hit your back
- Sit on a shower chair to rest while using birth ball and toilet throne techniques
- Use the shower rails for support during contractions
- Have your birth partner join you or provide support from outside the shower

Making Any Position Work for You

Regardless of which positions you try, keep these principles in mind: remember that changing your position may increase discomfort levels for a few contractions, so give each new position several contractions before evaluating its effectiveness. Pay attention to which positions feel intuitively right, practice position transitions before labor begins, and keep communicating with your birth team throughout the process. Most importantly, stay flexible—your needs may change as labor progresses.

Remember, your body and baby are working together in an intricate dance. It may take a few contractions to find your rhythm in a new position. Trust your instincts while staying open to suggestions from your experienced birth team. You may find that the best position for you is the one you least expected.

THE PUSHING PHASE: LISTENING TO YOUR BODY'S SIGNALS

When your labor progresses into the pushing phase, your positioning needs may change once again. While some women instinctively move into effective pushing positions, others benefit from guidance to find what works best. Remember, what feels right might surprise you. Remain open to your body's signals and your birth team's suggestions while drawing on these time-tested approaches.

Essential Pushing Positions

SIDE-LYING: REST WITHOUT SACRIFICING PROGRESS

When fatigue sets in, side-lying offers the perfect compromise between rest and effective positioning. This position:

- Helps prevent pelvic floor tearing
- Allows continued pelvic movement
- Gives your birth partner access to the hip and sacrum, allowing them to provide support through pressure
- Works well with or without an epidural

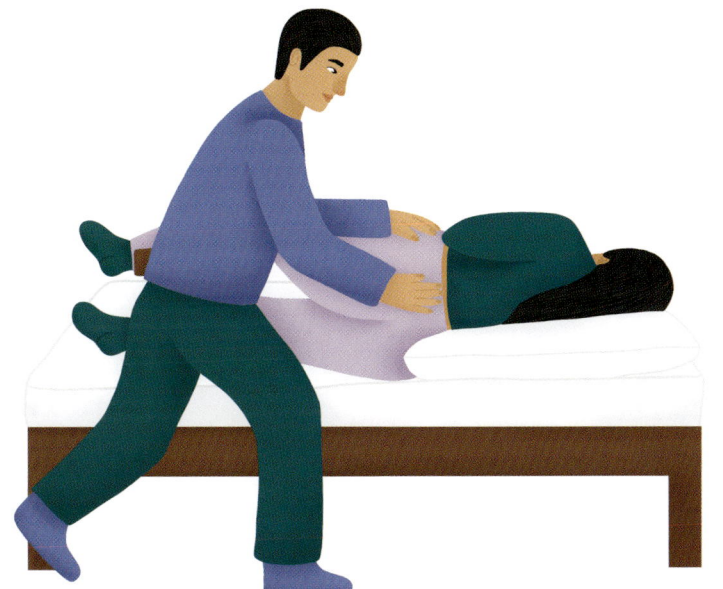

SIDE-LYING

- Provides good access for fetal monitoring
- Can be used during both the labor and delivery phases

MODIFIED HANDS AND KNEES

Getting on your hands and knees during the pushing phase offers several advantages. You can enhance the effectiveness of this position by:

- Pressing your hands firmly into the bed or floor
- Pulling your hands slightly toward your feet without moving your hands, as this naturally engages your core and supports your pushing efforts
- Rocking back and forth and moving your hips from side to side between contractions to encourage your baby's descent

- When using this position, your birth partner can provide invaluable support by applying pressure to your sacrum and hips.
- Can be used during both the labor and delivery phases

WIN-WIN POSITIONS FOR MONITORING

If your healthcare team requires better access to monitor your baby, place a pillow behind your back while side-lying. This partial side-lying position gives your medical team needed access while providing many benefits of true side-lying. Research shows side-lying can reduce pelvic floor tearing risk by 66.6 percent compared to other positions—allowing you to maintain protective advantages while accommodating monitoring needs.

Working with Different Birth Scenarios

Birth rarely follows a textbook pattern, and various situations may require different approaches. Let's explore how various positions can be adapted to common scenarios.

WHEN LABOR PROGRESSES QUICKLY

Sometimes labor moves faster than expected. While this might sound ideal, rapid labor can feel overwhelming and increase the risk of pelvic floor tearing. If this happens:

- Consider temporarily using positions that work against gravity
- Try getting on your elbows (or forearms) and knees, with your hips slightly higher than your shoulders
- Focus on your breathing to stay calm
- Work closely with your birth team to maintain control

WHEN YOUR BABY NEEDS HELP ENGAGING

If your baby isn't initially in the ideal position, don't worry—babies often adjust during labor, a phenomenon we sometimes call "baby acrobatics." To support this process:

- Try Child's Pose position while on your hands and knees.
- Experiment with asymmetrical positions, such as having one foot elevated on a stool.
- Give your baby time to respond to position changes.

- Communicate with your birth team about progress.

BREECH CONSIDERATIONS

If your baby is in a breech position (bottom or feet first), your position choices become even more important. Research suggests that lying on your right side as your baby crowns may help reduce pelvic floor tearing. However, always follow your healthcare team's guidance, as they'll help you find positions that:

- Support a safe descent
- Allow for optimal monitoring
- Allow for flexibility if they need to intervene
- Protect your pelvic floor

Putting It All Together

You now have the tools to feel confident throughout the birth process. We've discussed several strategies that can help you work with your body during contractions and the different stages of delivery, no matter how it unfolds. By choosing how you approach birth, you empower yourself to take control of your birth experience.

Remember, your five fundamental techniques for each contraction are:

- Pelvic floor relaxation
- Deep, low sounds
- Pelvic tilting
- Supportive pelvic pressure techniques
- Strategic positioning

LOOKING AHEAD: FROM BIRTH TO RECOVERY

As we conclude our exploration of birth positions and movement, it's important to remember that your journey doesn't end with delivery. Just as each phase of labor requires different positions and support, your fourth trimester will require its own kind of mindful movement and care.

The positions and movements you've learned in this chapter lay the foundation for your recovery journey. The body awareness you've developed, your understanding of pelvic movement, and the partnership you've built with your support team will serve you well as you navigate the postpartum period. Many of the principles we've discussed—listening to your body, moving with intention, and adapting to your needs—will be just as important during your postpartum recovery.

In the coming chapters we'll explore how to care for your body during the fourth trimester. You'll learn how to support your physical recovery, nurture your changing body, and gradually return to movement in ways that honor the remarkable journey you've completed.

THE FOURTH TRIMESTER AND BEYOND

Understanding Your Postpartum Body

Welcome to the fourth trimester—the first three months after your baby's arrival. This period represents a profound transition as you simultaneously heal from birth and adapt to the incredible demands of new motherhood. While much of the focus now shifts to your little one, we're here to support you. Our goal is to help you navigate recovery and adjust to life with your new baby.

The pressure to "bounce back" after pregnancy pervades our culture, but this mindset can hinder proper healing. Instead, embrace the concept of "nourish and flourish." Your body has accomplished something extraordinary—it's created, sustained, and birthed new life. Reward this accomplishment by allowing yourself the time and care needed to fully recover.

Recovery is different for everyone. Some days will feel like progress while others may bring unexpected challenges—and that's completely normal. Healing is a gradual, non-linear process. Focus on nurturing yourself and your baby during this important period, taking the time you need to recover and restore.

PHYSICAL CHANGES IN YOUR FOURTH TRIMESTER BODY

Over the course of forty weeks, your body underwent extraordinary changes in posture, strength, and function. While the first twelve weeks postpartum are essential for healing, your complete recovery journey may take longer and focusing only on the first twelve weeks is short-sighted. For instance, rebuilding vaginal muscle tone typically takes four to six months but may continue for up to a year. Similarly, your abdominal muscles need at least six months to rebuild their collagen structure and regain strength.

During these early months, you might experience muscle aches, urinary leakage during movement, or a feeling of pressure in your pelvic region. While these symptoms are common, they shouldn't become your new normal. With the right care and guidance, especially from a pelvic health specialist, you can navigate these challenges successfully.

Your Body's Early Recovery

The first six to eight weeks after birth are a time of profound natural healing. During this period your uterus gradually returns to its prepregnancy size, hormone levels shift and stabilize, and tissues begin to heal as fluid levels normalize. Meanwhile your joints, which became more mobile during pregnancy, start to regain stability.

During pregnancy your pelvis shifted to make space for your baby. You might notice your pelvis still tipping slightly forward, and this may affect your back and hips. This can lead to muscle and joint discomfort as your body realigns its posture and rebuilds core strength—a process that takes time. Changes in bladder control or sensations of pressure in your pelvic area are also common as your pelvic floor recovers from birth. Understanding these natural changes will help you protect your body during the demanding tasks of new parenthood.

BIRTH RECOVERY CARE

Your recovery timeline will be influenced by whether you had a vaginal or cesarean delivery. Embrace these changes as a testament to your strength and your journey into motherhood.

Vaginal Birth Recovery

If you delivered vaginally, your recovery may focus on perineal care and comfort measures. If approved by your healthcare team, gentle pelvic floor awareness exercises can support healing. Use perineal wash bottles to clean the area and pat it dry. Staying hydrated promotes tissue recovery, while taking sitz baths (a warm bath with or without Epsom salts for your perineum) and alternating ice and heat therapy can offer relief. Remember, pain management isn't just about comfort—it supports your overall healing process. You can read more about perineal care on page 144.

Cesarean Delivery Recovery

If you're recovering from a cesarean delivery, prioritize incision care and infection prevention. Keep the incision site clean and dry, following your healthcare team's instructions. Use pillows strategically when feeding your baby to protect your healing abdomen, and carefully follow lifting restrictions. If you were prescribed medications, take them as directed to manage discomfort and support healing. Remember a cesarean delivery is an abdominal surgery that requires adequate care to heal.

Protect your healing incision with these techniques:

For Coughing and Sneezing: Lift your head high and keep your throat open.

During Position Changes: Gently exhale during the most challenging part of the movement to reduce abdominal pressure. This technique is often referred to as "blow as you go" breathing.

Getting in and out of bed safely:

To get up:
- Bend your knees.
- Use a small bridge to reposition your hips away from the edge of the bed you are rolling toward.
- Roll onto your side with your knees bent.
- Push yourself up while looking down, keeping your knees angled toward the head of the bed.

To lie down:
- Sit with your knees angled toward the head of the bed.
- Cross your ankles.
- Look down and lower yourself onto your elbows while lifting your feet onto the bed.

- Roll onto your back from your side, keeping your knees bent.
- Bridge if you need to reposition to the center of the bed.

Scar Tissue Mobilization

Whether from a cesarean delivery or vaginal birth, your incision or lacerations require proper care to promote optimal healing.

During the first six weeks postpartum, focus on gentle awareness. Start by resting your hand near the scar to begin familiarizing yourself with it. As you feel ready, gradually progress to looking at the scar and gently touching it. If the area is sensitive, try using the back of your hand or a soft material, such as a light scarf, for a gentler touch.

Once your incision is fully healed— typically after six weeks—you can begin more active scar mobilization. Regardless of whether you've experienced a perineal tear or had an abdominal incision, you can mobilize the scar tissue to reduce pain, improve its movement, and desensitize the area.

INITIAL SCAR MOBILIZATION

- Place your fingers half an inch to an inch away from the scar.
- Apply gentle pressure without sliding your fingers around.
- Make small movements, such as side-to-side, up-and-down, or circular motions.

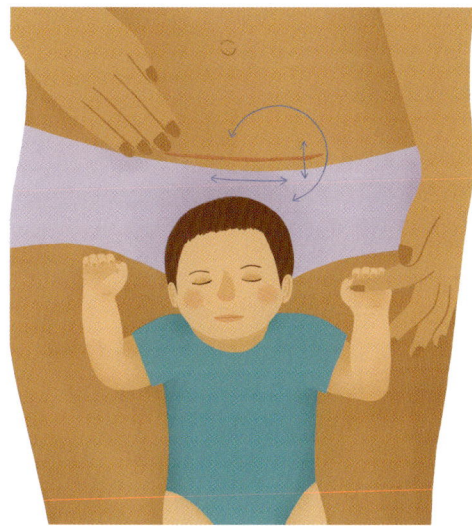

- Spend about 30 seconds on each area.
- Gradually move closer to the scar.
- Keep your sessions brief (3 to 5 minutes daily).
- Finish by gently massaging lotion or vitamin E oil into the scar.

ADVANCED SCAR MOBILIZATION TECHNIQUES

- Pinch and lift the incision.
- Stretch the skin along the incision by gently pulling it from one side while holding down on the other side.
- Practice lifting and moving the tissue up and down.

IMPORTANT NOTES

- Stop if the scar becomes red or inflamed.
- Watch for any openings.
- Use sunscreen on exposed scars (after the wound has fully healed).
- Consult your healthcare team if the scar raises or remains painful.

EMBRACING YOUR OWN BIRTH EXPERIENCE & RECOVERY

No matter how you brought your baby into this world, your delivery and path to healing are unique. In creating life your body has accomplished something extraordinary.

During the postpartum period, each body undergoes the same fundamental changes, regardless of how you gave birth. These universal experiences include hormonal shifts that support healing and milk production, postural adaptations as your body returns to its non-pregnant state, and the emotional transition into motherhood. If you're among the one in five mothers who had a cesarean delivery, you will also need additional care instructions for your abdominal incision. Using the term cesarean delivery, rather than "C-section" can be a powerful way to embrace and validate your delivery experience.

Your birth team will provide instructions based on your delivery type, but the core principle remains the same: Your body has immediate healing capabilities. Strengthening your core will be invaluable in your overall recovery no matter how you gave birth, but the timeline for resuming normal everyday activities, core-focused strengthening, and then high-level cardiovascular routines will depend on your birth experience. Instead of comparing your recovery timeline to others or to preconceived expectations, focus on following your healthcare team's guidance and tuning in to your body's needs.

Remember, whether you're caring for a perineal tear or an abdominal incision, these marks of motherhood tell the story of how you brought your baby into the world.

MANAGING YOUR DAILY ENERGY

Your recovery involves more than just physical healing—it requires careful management of your energy reserves.

FROM THE PRO
Jessica's Energy Insights

Many new mothers feel pressured to return to their pre-baby activity levels, but it's helpful to think of your energy as a daily budget that needs careful management. Some days, you'll wake up ready to tackle the world; other days, you may need extra rest—and both are completely valid. Instead of pushing through fatigue, learn to work with your energy patterns. This self-care practice will serve you well throughout motherhood.

EARLY MOVEMENT GUIDELINES

Movement during early recovery isn't about fitness—it's about gently supporting your body's healing process and maintaining basic function. While Chapter 18 gives detailed movement guidance, these first weeks will lay the groundwork for your return to activity.

- **Weeks Zero to Two:** Prioritize rest and recovery. Gently walking around your home or taking a short outdoor stroll can help promote circulation. Start gentle whole core and pelvic floor activations from Chapters 18 and 19.
- **Weeks Two to Four:** Gradually increase how long you walk and add light household activities while maintaining core and pelvic floor awareness.
- **Weeks Four to Six:** Many women can begin more regular activities and guided exercises once approved by their healthcare team.

BUILDING YOUR SUPPORT NETWORK

Recovery thrives with support. Consider who you'd like to have on your recovery team in addition to your healthcare providers. Your loved ones likely want to help but might not know how.

Clear communication is key. Be specific about what kind of support you need, whether it's meal preparation, household tasks, baby care to enable your physical healing or exercise program, or simply quiet company. When setting boundaries around visits and help, think of it as protecting your healing environment. Create a clear plan for both hospital and home visits that prioritizes your need for rest and bonding.

Remember, setting clear boundaries isn't selfish—it's vital for your recovery and your baby's well-being.

BABY BLUES, POSTPARTUM DEPRESSION & RECOVERY

While the joys of parenthood are profound, the postpartum period brings significant emotional changes. Most new parents experience what's commonly known as the "baby blues" during the first two weeks after birth. Symptoms may include mild mood swings, occasional tearfulness, and feeling overwhelmed by new responsibilities. These feelings typically peak around day five and resolve naturally as your hormones stabilize and you adjust to your new role.

However, if emotional challenges persist beyond two weeks or become more intense, you may be experiencing postpartum depression. Symptoms can include persistent sadness, difficulty bonding with your baby, overwhelming fatigue, and withdrawal from family and friends.

Research has shown a significant link between pelvic floor disorders, such as urinary incontinence, and an increased risk of developing postpartum depression by three-fold. This connection underscores the need to address pelvic health as part of comprehensive postnatal care. Physical discomfort and the functional limitations from pelvic floor dysfunction can impact your sense of well-being and contribute to emotional distress.

Physical activity serves as a protective factor against mood disorders for many women, but should be thoughtfully implemented during recovery. The endorphins released during appropriate movement can help regulate mood and reduce symptoms of depression and anxiety. This is another important reason to approach your physical recovery with intention rather than rushing the process.

Remember, postpartum depression is more common than most people realize and can begin during pregnancy or after birth. It's not a reflection of your abilities as a parent, and it usually responds well to professional treatment.

If you're concerned about your emotional well-being, validated tools like the Edinburgh Postnatal Depression Scale and the City Birth Trauma Scale can help you assess your symptoms and decide when to seek support.

These questionnaires can be a starting point for discussions with your healthcare team.

Your emotional well-being deserves as much attention as your physical recovery. There are many resources available to support you, including mothers' groups, postpartum doulas, and mental health professionals who specialize in postpartum care. If you experience persistent symptoms or have thoughts of harming yourself or your baby, reach out to your healthcare provider immediately. In the United States, you can contact the 988 Suicide & Crisis Lifeline for 24/7 support.

Remember, seeking help isn't just about you—it's about creating the healthiest environment for both you and your baby.

LOOKING FORWARD: YOUR CONTINUED RECOVERY

As you move through your first few postpartum weeks, you'll likely notice patterns in your recovery, physical symptoms, sleep, and energy reserves. Some days, you will experience noticeable progress, while others might feel like a step backward.

In Chapter 17, we'll explore how to apply recovery principles—especially sleep, energy reserves, lifting mechanics, rest—to your daily life with your newborn, creating routines that honor both your healing needs and your new responsibilities.

Following that, Chapter 18 will take an in-depth look at pelvic floor health and introduce a structured program designed to rebuild your foundation from the inside out. You'll learn techniques and exercises specifically designed to restore pelvic floor function, rebuild core strength, and support your return to the activities you love—all while respecting your body's natural recovery timeline.

CHAPTER 17

Integrating Recovery with Daily Baby Care

The fourth trimester presents a delicate balance: healing your body while caring for your newborn. In Chapter 16, we explored the foundations of your recovery journey and the physiological changes happening in your postpartum body. In this chapter, we'll explore how daily activities with your baby affect your healing tissues, hormonal balance, and energy systems—empowering you to make choices that support your return to strength.

FEEDING YOUR BABY: IMPACT ON YOUR PHYSICAL RECOVERY

Whether nursing or formula feeding, your feeding choice significantly influences your body's recovery process. Understanding these effects empowers you to make informed decisions that support your healing journey.

How Nursing Benefits Mom & Baby

Nursing offers significant benefits for both mother and baby. First and foremost, for mothers, nursing can support postpartum weight management and may lower the risk of breast cancer. It may also improve abdominal tone and promote nerve healing in your physical recovery. For babies, nursing helps build their immune system during the first 4 to 6 weeks, reduces the risk of sudden infant death syndrome, and provides easily digestible nourishment.

How Nursing Affects Your Recovery

If you choose to nurse, your body undergoes specific physiological changes that directly impact your recovery timeline. The hormone oxytocin released during nursing helps your uterus contract back to prepregnancy size more efficiently, potentially speeding up this aspect of recovery. However, nursing also creates higher caloric needs (about 500 extra calories daily) and can influence your sleep patterns, both of which affect your overall healing.

Understanding these influences allows you to work with—rather than against—your nursing body during recovery.

Nursing Support

Many new mothers worry about their baby getting enough milk. Remember that you and your baby are learning a new skill together—one that requires patience and support. It's normal for your milk supply to take time to establish itself during this learning period.

Milk supply is regulated by oxytocin and bonding: your baby's feeding patterns signal your body to produce the right amount of milk. This demand-supply relationship is key to establishing a healthy feeding routine. In general, it's recommended to avoid pumping during the early days to help your body regulate milk supply based on your baby's needs.

Regular, effective feeding sessions not only regulate your milk production but also help prevent complications like clogged ducts. Offering both breasts during each feeding and staying well-hydrated and properly nourished supports your milk supply while meeting your body's increased recovery needs.

If you do experience clogged ducts, check whether your sports bra might be too compressive. A pelvic health physiotherapist is trained to provide treatment for clogged ducts as part of your overall recovery care. For a small percentage of mothers, more serious complications like mastitis may develop, indicated by redness, inflammation, flu-like symptoms, fever, unusual fatigue, and persistent clogged ducts—all requiring prompt medical attention.

A lactation consultant can provide invaluable support for your nursing journey, offering guidance on everything from nutrition and proper hydration to positioning techniques and feeding schedules that complement your recovery goals. They can help you establish routines that support both your baby's needs and your body's healing.

FROM THE PRO
Jessica's Insight on the Role of Oxytocin and Bonding

When nursing, the release of oxytocin does more than support milk production and help your uterus return to its prepregnancy size: it promotes bonding with your baby. Try to stay present during these feeding moments rather than multitasking when possible. While multitasking might be necessary for many mothers, it can potentially impact your milk supply if you're experiencing challenges.

Formula Feeding: Benefits to Recovery

If you're using formula, whether exclusively or as a supplement, this choice offers specific advantages for your physical recovery. The predictable feeding schedule can allow for more consolidated sleep, which is critical for tissue repair and hormone regulation. Formula feeding also allows others to participate in feeding, giving you dedicated time for recovery practices or simply rest.

If you need medications, have dietary restrictions, or experience challenges with milk supply, formula feeding provides flexibility in caring for your body's needs during recovery.

While some women choose to formula feed for their training schedules, remember that currently the World Health Organization recommends exclusively feeding infants milk from the mother for the first six months, followed by the gradual introduction of complementary foods while continuing to nurse for two years or more. While it isn't always possible, it's important to feel informed and empowered when making your parenting choices.

Exercise and Nursing

For mothers who plan to return to regular physical activity while nursing, timing is key. Your breasts will likely feel fuller in the morning, which generally makes afternoon exercise more comfortable.

When possible, plan to feed your baby before exercising. This can make your breasts feel lighter and allow you to move more comfortably. A supportive sports bra is essential to protect sensitive breast tissue, but avoid choosing one that compresses too tightly, as this could lead to blocked ducts.

Your body needs extra fluids for both feeding and exercise, so be sure to stay well-hydrated, especially in warm weather. Be mindful of your energy levels during your workouts, as they may fluctuate more than you expect. Remember, producing milk burns a significant amount of calories, so it's a good idea to have a light meal before exercising and to pack snacks to keep your energy up throughout your activity.

Most importantly, take comfort in knowing that moderate exercise won't affect your milk production or quality. Your body is remarkably capable of supporting both your recovery and your baby's needs.

FROM THE PRO
Shannon on Nursing and Physical Recovery

After I gave birth, I was committed to nursing my baby, but because I was still competing in Track & Field, I also needed to return to training and racing quickly. The logistics were complicated, and the consensus in my industry was that nursing and athletics couldn't coexist.

As I juggled both new parenthood and professional demands, I reminded myself that my daughter didn't ask to be born; I chose to have her. While having a child complicated life immeasurably, it gave me a new perspective and conviction I'd never known. When others tried to dictate how I should parent, my determination to forge my own path only strengthened.

How did I balance nursing and physical activity? Through the same detailed planning and committed effort that had always supported my demanding training schedule. I chose a mobile pump that allowed me to multitask—eating breakfast or doing morning stretches while pumping. My milk went directly into bottles, minimizing cleanup and simplifying childcare handoffs. By streamlining this process, I only needed to wake 30 minutes earlier—with a structured plan, it was manageable.

Pumping before training meant lighter breasts during workouts, improving my biomechanics. Since I'd already burned significant calories, I was vigilant about fueling properly with a good breakfast and packing fluids and electrolytes to support muscle function. I desperately wished for research on optimal nutrition for nursing athletes, but lacking that, I prepared thoroughly and listened to my body's signals.

I ate my packed lunch immediately after workouts, taking advantage of the crucial 45 to 60 minute recovery window—a practice I'd started before having children. This timing proved essential because my daughter typically needed to nurse as soon as I arrived home, and postponing nutrition would have compromised my recovery.

Surprisingly, I looked forward to nursing after training. Though exhausted, nursing provided exactly what I needed—a moment to disconnect from external demands and be fully present. Like finding mental clarity during a run, I could let my thoughts wander while holding my daughter. The combination of exercise followed by nursing gave me a double dose of oxytocin, creating profound joy that actually enhanced my recovery.

The results spoke for themselves: while still nursing, I ran Olympic qualifying times in both the 1500m and 5000m. My 5000m performance ranked eleventh globally that season and set a US Masters record at age thirty-five—clear evidence that nursing and athletic excellence can coexist.

My advice from this experience: Always remember your choices are your own, and if anyone claims you can't be strong as a mother while choosing to nurse, simply tell them, "Watch me!"

PHYSICAL INTIMACY AND RECOVERY AFTER BIRTH

Sexual intimacy undergoes significant changes during the postpartum period as your body heals. These changes are driven by both physical recovery needs and hormonal factors, particularly for nursing mothers.

The hormones involved in milk production create specific challenges for intercourse. Estrogen levels naturally remain lower while nursing, which can affect vaginal tissue health, lubrication, and flexibility. While fatigue can impact intimacy, so can nursing. Nursing also increases prolactin levels, which is essential for milk production but may temporarily reduce libido as your body prioritizes infant care.

The oxytocin released during nursing provides a sense of contentment in bonding with your baby, while lower testosterone levels may temporarily decrease desire for physical intimacy. These hormonal shifts serve an evolutionary purpose but can create challenges for couples.

Although these changes can feel significant, they're temporary and don't predict your long-term sexual satisfaction—regardless of your birth experience. Open communication with your partner about your body's healing needs creates the foundation for maintaining connection during this transition. Make sure to discuss any persistent discomfort with your healthcare provider.

When you're ready to resume intimate relations, consider these recovery-supportive approaches:

- Use water-based lubricants to improve your comfort.
- Apply lubricant externally, internally, and encourage your partner to use it as well.
- Explore positions that give you control over depth and pressure on your healing tissues.
- Initially, choose positions that allow you to guide penetration.
- Set aside at least 20 to 30 minutes to allow for proper arousal and relaxation.
- Communicate openly about what feels comfortable for your healing body.

Remember that intimacy encompasses more than intercourse. During your recovery, exploring alternative forms of connection—sensual massage, kissing, cuddling—can help maintain your bond while respecting your body's healing timeline.

HOW BABY CARE AFFECTS YOUR RECOVERY

Each time you lift, carry, feed, or soothe your baby, you have an opportunity establish and reinforce movement patterns. While these movements may seem simple, they occur dozens of times daily and cumulatively create new habits. Proper postures and movement patterns during these frequent activities allow you to transform routine baby care into opportunities to rebuild functional strength while protecting vulnerable tissues.

Daily Baby Care Movement Guidelines

WHEN FEEDING YOUR BABY

- Use supportive pillows to bring your baby to breast/bottle height.
- Maintain neutral spine alignment rather than hunching forward.
- Keep a footstool nearby to maintain optimal pelvic positioning.
- Tuck your chin slightly when looking down to protect your neck.
- Change positions regularly during longer feeding sessions.
- Keep hydration and other essentials within easy reach to avoid having to twist.

WHEN LIFTING YOUR BABY

- Stand close to the crib or changing table in a staggered stance.
- Activate your whole core before bending.
- Bend your knees to reduce hinging at your back.
- Exhale gently on exertion to manage intra-abdominal pressure.
- Use your leg strength rather than back muscles.
- Keep your baby close to your body's center of gravity during the lift.

WHEN CARRYING YOUR BABY

- Alternate sides regularly or carry your baby in front to balance muscular development.
- Choose properly-fitting carriers that distribute weight evenly across your shoulders and hips.
- Maintain proper alignment without compensatory patterns (arching your back, or, shrugging).
- Take regular breaks to reset your posture and relieve pressure.
- Avoid single-shoulder diaper bags that create uneven loading.
- Consider backpack-style bags for even weight distribution.
- Use a stroller to help carry the car seat whenever possible.

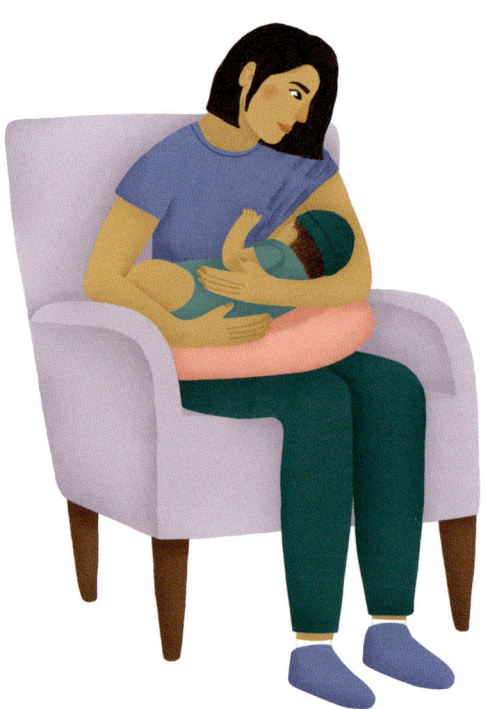

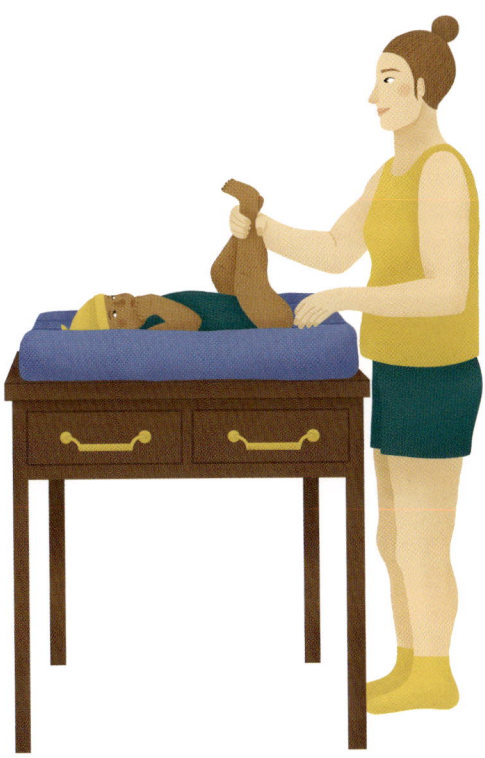

WHEN SOOTHING YOUR BABY

- Make bouncing movements by bending your knees versus from your back.
- Use "shushing" sounds which help core activation and calm your baby.
- Practice maintaining neutral pelvis during standing motions.
- Bounce on a therapy ball to engage stabilizing muscles.
- Integrate gentle lunges in several directions to maintain lower body strength.

WHEN BATHING YOUR BABY

- Use a portable tub at counter height when possible.
- Kneel beside a bathtub rather than bending over.
- Keep supplies within easy reach to avoid having to twist.
- Use a non-slip pad for safety and stability.
- Rest one foot on a small stool when standing at the sink to relieve back pressure.

WHEN CHANGING DIAPERS

- Position changing stations at hip height to prevent bending.
- Keep supplies organized and within arm's reach.
- Stand close to the changing surface to avoid having to lean or reach
- Kneel rather than bend when using a low surface.
- Consider multiple changing stations to minimize carrying between floors.

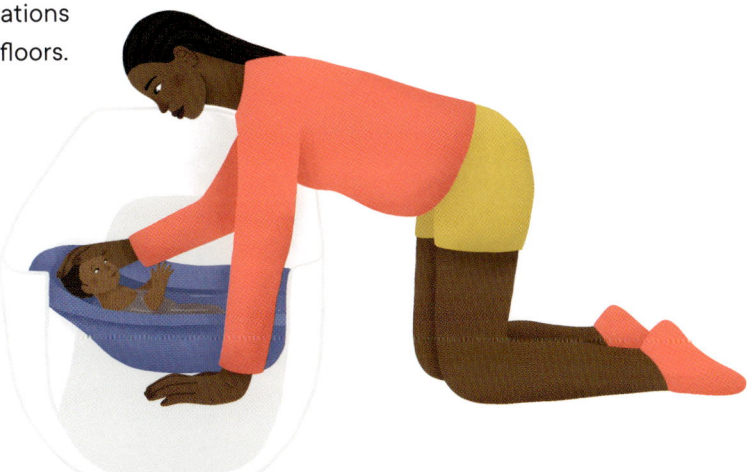

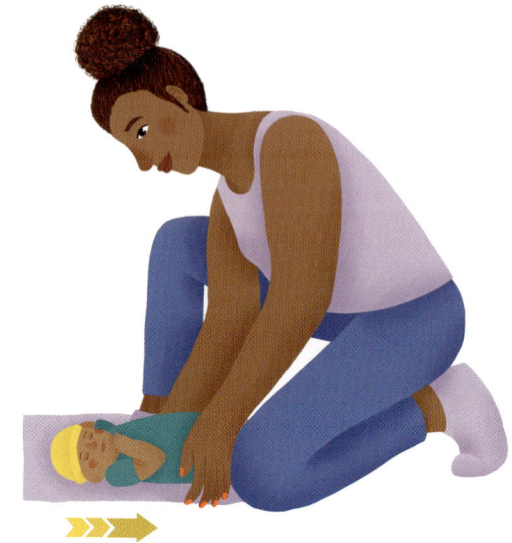

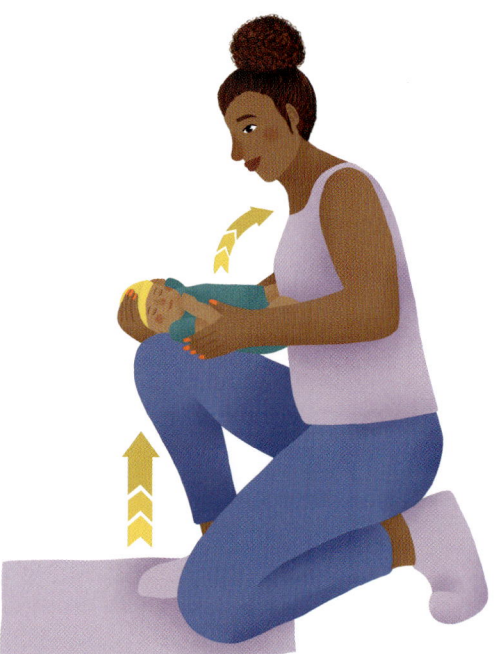

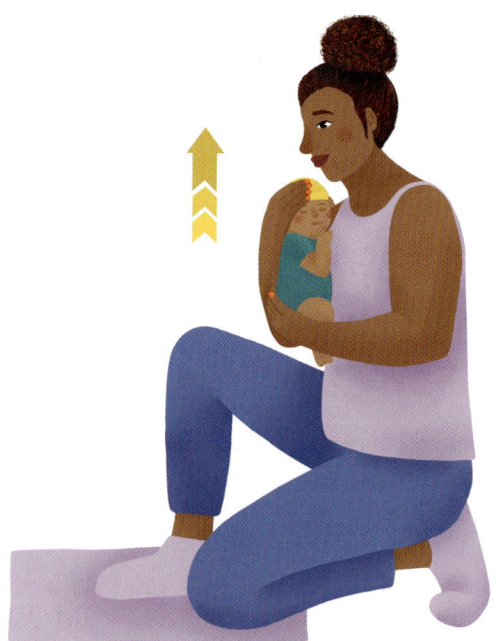

- Keep your palms flat to avoid wrist issues.
- Use supportive pillows so you can relax your arm muscles.
- Avoid shrugging your shoulders toward your ears which creates neck tension.
- Engage your shoulder blades gently down and in towards your bra line for postural activation.

DURING FLOOR TIME WITH YOUR BABY

- Sit with your back against furniture or a wall for support.
- Roll to your side before getting up from the floor if you've had a cesarean delivery.

These mindful movement strategies protect your healing tissues while supporting the gradual restoration of functional strength and movement patterns.

SLEEP: THE FOUNDATION OF RECOVERY

Sleep is your body's most powerful recovery tool. During sleep, your body releases growth hormone, repairs muscles and tissues, regulates hormones and reduces inflammation, replenishes energy stores and immunity, and consolidates neural pathways essential for regaining functional movement.

Research shows that even moderate sleep deprivation can delay wound healing by up to 60% and increase inflammatory markers throughout the body. Research also shows that athletes who consistently get less than eight hours of sleep double their risk of injury. This is largely because sleep deprivation reduces the synthesis of muscle. Sleep deprivation can also affect your muscles' ability to produce protein and reduces their overall strength capacity. Keep this in mind as you decide how much weight to use for your exercise program in the next months.

While continuous sleep is rarely possible with a newborn, the quality of sleep you do get significantly impacts recovery. Brief periods of deep sleep provide more restorative benefits than longer periods of fragmented sleep. Sleeping when baby sleeps and arranging night shifts that give you the largest quantity of quality sleep can be paramount in your recovery. By prioritizing sleep quality whenever possible, you may accelerate your overall recovery more effectively than through many other interventions.

PARTNER COMMUNICATION AND RECOVERY SUPPORT

Your partner plays a crucial role in supporting your physical recovery. Have direct conversations about specific ways they can help protect your recovering tissues rather than assuming they understand your needs.

Be explicit about activities that cause discomfort, and identify concrete ways your partner can assist with physically demanding tasks. Frame these conversations around your shared goal of optimal healing.

Since sleep deprivation significantly impacts tissue healing, work together to divide nighttime responsibilities in a way that supports your recovery through adequate rest periods. Clear communication about your physical needs isn't selfish—it's essential for creating an environment where recovery can flourish alongside new parenthood.

LOOKING FORWARD: *Your Continuing Recovery Journey Pelvic Floor Rehabilitation*

As you integrate these principles into your daily care routine with your baby, you're establishing patterns that support long-term healing and strength. By understanding how feeding choices, sleep patterns, and everyday movements affect your healing tissues, you empower yourself to make small but significant adjustments that honor your recovery needs alongside your new responsibilities.

In our next chapter, we'll explore specific rehabilitation approaches for your pelvic floor, which forms the foundation of your core strength. You'll learn targeted exercises and techniques designed to restore proper function to this crucial muscle group. Then, in Chapter 19, we will guide you through a progressive 12-week training program to systematically rebuild strength from your core outward, respecting your body's specific healing timeline. You can use Chapters 18, 19, and 20 in tandem as each follow the 12-week timeline.

Your Pelvic Floor Rehabilitation

The postpartum period brings significant changes to your pelvic floor. In fact, about 50 percent of women experience noticeable changes in this area. Whether you had an episiotomy, experienced natural tearing during delivery, or had no tearing at all, your pelvic floor needs time to heal and restore. During the first weeks of your postpartum period, you'll likely notice substantial improvements as your body's collagen makeup shifts in response to hormonal changes, supporting the healing process.

FROM THE PRO
Jessica's Perspective on Recovery

Think of your pelvic floor as part of an integrated support system. The fascia supporting your organs, along with your hips, back, and abdominal muscles, work together to stabilize your pelvis. After pregnancy and birth, this system needs time to recalibrate.

RECOVERY: TIMELINE, EXPECTATIONS, AND BEST PRACTICES

Postpartum symptoms, such as occasional leakage or a sense of pelvic pressure, are common, but they shouldn't become your permanent normal. After a vaginal birth, the pelvic floor muscles typically take four to six months to regain optimal tone, although this process may take up to a year. This variation is entirely normal—your body is taking the time it needs to heal.

The Hormone Factor

Estrogen plays a vital role in your postpartum recovery, especially when it comes to your pelvic floor. This important hormone helps keep your pelvic floor muscles and urinary tract tissues optimal in strength and function. After childbirth, particularly if you're nursing, your estrogen levels naturally drop as your body prioritizes milk production.

Estrogen supports your pelvic floor by strengthening your muscles and bulking up the urethra while improving vaginal tissue lubrication. During this time of lower estrogen, you might notice increased urinary leakage, changes in muscle function, and reduced sensations during intercourse.

FROM THE PRO
Jessica's Hormone Insight

Knowing the role hormones play in your body can help you understand why some aspects of incontinence recovery might take longer if you're nursing. This doesn't mean you're not healing—it simply means that your body is prioritizing milk production over thickening of the urethra. This temporary trade-off is natural and should resolve as your hormones gradually return to their non-pregnancy levels.

Managing Early Postpartum Challenges and Discomfort

PERINEAL CARE

If you had a vaginal delivery or attempted one, it's important to care for your perineum with effective strategies for managing discomfort. Ice therapy can provide significant relief when applied every two hours for 10-15 minutes during the first few days postpartum.

You can create comfortable, anatomically shaped ice packs by pouring water over a sanitary pad or baby diaper, then shaping it over a bowl before freezing. Remember to wrap ice packs in a towel or cloth before use to avoid placing them directly on your skin, which could cause tissue damage.

Additional Comfort Measures
- Use lidocaine spray (if approved by your healthcare team).
- Try medicated cooling pads.
- Support the perineum with gentle pressure if you need to cough, sneeze, or exert yourself.

GENTLE VULVAR CARE

Taking proper care of your vulva is important throughout your life, but it's especially important postpartum due to pelvic lacerations and reduced estrogen levels. Here are some ways to help support the natural healing process.

Cleansing and Comfort
- Clean external areas only—your vagina naturally cleans itself.
- Trim pubic hair but do not shave it as hair is important to wick away moisture.
- Use unscented cleaning products designed for sensitive skin.
- Choose loose-fitting, breathable cotton clothing.
- Wash garments with fragrance-free, sensitive-skin detergent.

Monitoring Your Health

- Be mindful of any discomfort, sensitivity, or changes in discharge color or smell that might indicate infection. The postpartum estrogen drop can affect vaginal pH values and benefit bacteria. Contact your healthcare provider if you notice significant changes, as early attention supports optimal healing.

MANAGING HEMORRHOIDS

Hemorrhoids are a common part of the childbirth process and affect about 40 percent of women. While uncomfortable and sometimes painful, they're typically harmless and resolve within days to weeks after delivery. Hemorrhoids develop due to restricted blood flow in the anal region and natural straining during the pushing phase of labor.

You might have hemorrhoids if you:

- Find it painful or difficult to sit.
- Notice bright red blood when wiping after bowel movements.
- Feel a small lump near your anus.
- Experience itching or pain around the anal area.

Relief Strategies

Use gravity to your advantage and gently care for your anal area to help manage discomfort.

Position and Movement

- Rest on your side or stomach to reduce pressure.
- Avoid prolonged sitting whenever possible.
- Move gently but regularly to promote circulation.

Bathroom Habits

- Avoid straining during bowel movements.
- Use stool softeners as recommended by your healthcare provider.
- Choose foods that help prevent constipation.
- Clean the anal area gently using a perineal wash bottle.
- Pat yourself dry instead of wiping.

Comfort Measures

- Apply ice (with a protective layer) for 10–15 minutes at a time.
- Use medicated pads or witch hazel.
- Soak in warm Epsom salt baths.
- Try over-the-counter creams that are approved by your healthcare team.

BOWEL HEALTH

Your first postpartum bowel movement can be anxiety-inducing, especially if you've had an epidural or experienced tearing during delivery. Your pelvic area houses several organs, so when constipation creates fullness in your bowel, which then takes up more space, it directly affects your bladder. In short, the pressure from constipation can place additional strain on your bladder.

Managing your bowel health is an essential part of your overall pelvic floor recovery, as constipation often contributes to urinary leakage.

We'll share some strategies that can help support healthy bowel function below.

Natural Support Strategies

- Start your day with warm liquids to stimulate your intestines.
- Eat breakfast to activate your digestive system.
- Ensure a balanced mix of insoluble and soluble fiber in your diet. Good sources include stone fruits (especially prunes) and chia seeds.
- Consult your healthcare provider about any medication you may need.

MANAGING BOWEL MOVEMENTS DURING POSTPARTUM RECOVERY

- Position yourself with your feet flat on the floor (use a small footstool if needed).
- Lean slightly forward.
- Support your perineum with a clean washcloth or your hand.
- When you go to the bathroom, use the breathing techniques you've learned. Let your belly expand and your anus relax, then gently tighten your abdominals.
- Avoid straining.
- Clean the anal area gently with a perineal wash bottle when you're done.
- Pat dry carefully.

Note: In some cases, leaning backward during bowel movements may be more beneficial. If this applies to you, it's worth discussing with your healthcare team.

Birth Control Management

Around 6-8 weeks postpartum, your healthcare provider will likely discuss birth control options, as fertility can return before your menstrual cycle. Because different types of birth control impact your recovery and ability to monitor your energy reserves, consider sharing the following information with your healthcare provider to help create the most appropriate plan for your needs:

- Previous menstrual symptoms and pain
- Emotional well-being
- Family planning preferences
- Migraine history (if applicable)
- Future exercise goals

From an exercise perspective, it's important to recognize that using certain birth control may impact your menstrual cycle. As a result, monitoring for RED-S becomes more challenging since a regular monthly period is an important indicator of your overall health. To check into potential RED-S symptoms, please visit page 26.

Your Thirty-Day Strong as a Mother Recovery Program

You can begin gentle pelvic floor exercises as soon as you feel ready after childbirth—even during your hospital stay if you don't have a catheter. While doing these exercises on your own offers about a 9 to 17 percent success rate in resolving issues such as urinary leakage, working with a pelvic floor specialist increases success rates to 60 to 75 percent. If you need additional support, consider professional guidance, which can be invaluable in your recovery.

Your thirty-day *Strong as a Mother* recovery program is designed to progressively build pelvic floor strength and function. If you need to refresh your memory on proper technique, revisit Foundational Pelvic Floor Exercises on pages 204-205.

Note: Perform all Static Holds exercise at 30 to 50 percent of your strength throughout the program.

Week One

DAY ONE

Rest, shower, and celebrate your body's incredible achievement.

DAY TWO

Continue resting and celebrating.

DAY THREE

Practice gentle pelvic floor activation by contracting your pelvic floor muscles with 30 to 50 percent strength during sit-to-stand movements throughout the day.

DAY FOUR

Continue practicing gentle pelvic floor activation by contracting your pelvic floor muscles with 30 to 50 percent strength during sit-to-stand movements throughout the day.

DAY FIVE

- **Static Holds:** 5 seconds, 5 reps
- **Quick Flicks:** 5 reps
- **Elevator Exercises:** 5 reps
- **Half-Holds with 3 Quick Flicks:** 5 reps

DAY SIX

- **Static Holds:** 5 seconds, 5 reps
- **Quick Flicks:** 5 reps
- **Elevator Exercises:** 5 reps
- **Half-Holds with 3 Quick Flicks:** 5 reps

- **Static Holds:** 5 seconds, 5 reps
- **Quick Flicks:** 5 reps
- **Elevator Exercises:** 5 reps
- **Half-Holds with 3 Quick Flicks:** 5 reps

Week Two

DAY EIGHT

- **Static Holds:** 5 seconds, 8 reps
- **Quick Flicks:** 10 reps
- **Elevator Exercises:** 10 reps
- **Half-Holds with 3 Quick Flicks:** 10 reps

DAY NINE

- **Static Holds:** 5 seconds, 10 reps
- **Quick Flicks:** 10 reps
- **Elevator Exercises:** 10 reps
- **Half-Holds with 3 Quick Flicks:** 10 reps

DAY TEN

- **Static Holds:** 5 seconds, 10 reps
- **Quick Flicks:** 10 reps
- **Elevator Exercises:** 10 reps
- **Half-Holds with 3 Quick Flicks:** 10 reps

DAY ELEVEN

- **Static Holds:** 8 seconds, 5 reps
- **Quick Flicks:** 10 reps
- **Elevator Exercises:** 10 reps
- **Half-Holds with 3 Quick Flicks:** 10 reps

DAY TWELVE

- **Static Holds:** 8 seconds, 5 reps
- **Quick Flicks:** 10 reps
- **Elevator Exercises:** 10 reps
- **Half-Holds with 3 Quick Flicks:** 10 reps

DAY THIRTEEN

- **Static Holds:** 8 seconds, 8 reps
- **Quick Flicks:** 10 reps
- **Elevator Exercises:** 10 reps
- **Half-Holds with 3 Quick Flicks:** 10 reps

DAY FOURTEEN

- **Static Holds:** 8 seconds, 8 reps
- **Quick Flicks:** 10 reps
- **Elevator Exercises:** 10 reps
- **Half-Holds with 3 Quick Flicks:** 10 reps

Week Three

DAY FIFTEEN

- **Static Holds:** 8 seconds, 10 reps
- **Quick Flicks:** 15 reps
- **Elevator Exercises:** 10 reps
- **Half-Holds with 3 Quick Flicks:** 15 reps

DAY SIXTEEN

- **Static Holds:** 8 seconds, 10 reps
- **Quick Flicks:** 15 reps
- **Elevator Exercises:** 10 reps
- **Half-Holds with 3 Quick Flicks:** 15 reps

DAY SEVENTEEN

- **Static Holds:** 10 seconds, 5 reps
- **Quick Flicks:** 15 reps
- **Elevator Exercises:** 10 reps
- **Half-Holds with 3 Quick Flicks:** 15 reps

DAY EIGHTEEN

- **Static Holds:** 10 seconds, 5 reps
- **Quick Flicks:** 15 reps
- **Elevator Exercises:** 10 reps
- **Half-Holds with 3 Quick Flicks:** 15 reps

DAY NINETEEN

- **Static Holds:** 10 seconds, 8 reps
- **Quick Flicks:** 15 reps
- **Elevator Exercises:** 10 reps
- **Half-Holds with 3 Quick Flicks:** 15 reps

DAY TWENTY

- **Static Holds:** 10 seconds, 8 reps
- **Quick Flicks:** 15 reps
- **Elevator Exercises:** 10 reps
- **Half-Holds with 3 Quick Flicks:** 15 reps

DAY TWENTY-ONE

- **Static Holds:** 10 seconds, 10 reps
- **Quick Flicks:** 15 reps
- **Elevator Exercises:** 10 reps
- **Half-Holds with 3 Quick Flicks:** 15 reps

Week Four

DAY TWENTY-TWO

- **Static Holds:** 10 seconds, 10 reps
- **Quick Flicks:** 20 repetitions
- **Elevator Exercises:** 10 repetitions
- **Half-Holds with 3 Quick Flicks:** 20 reps

DAY TWENTY-THREE

- **Static Holds:** 15 seconds, 5 reps
- **Quick Flicks:** 20 reps
- **Elevator Exercises:** 10 reps
- **Half-Holds with 3 Quick Flicks:** 20 reps

DAY TWENTY-FOUR

- **Static Holds:** 15 seconds, 5 reps
- **Quick Flicks:** 20 reps
- **Elevator Exercises:** 10 reps
- **Half-Holds with 3 Quick Flicks:** 20 reps

DAY TWENTY-FIVE

- **Static Holds:** 20 seconds, 4 reps
- **Quick Flicks:** 20 reps
- **Elevator Exercises:** 10 reps
- **Half-Holds with 3 Quick Flicks:** 20 reps

DAY TWENTY-SIX

- **Static Holds:** 20 seconds, 4 reps
- **Quick Flicks:** 20 reps
- **Elevator Exercises:** 10 reps
- **Half-Holds with 3 Quick Flicks:** 20 reps

DAY TWENTY-SEVEN

- **Static Holds:** 25 seconds, 3 reps
- **Quick Flicks:** 20 reps
- **Elevator Exercises:** 10 reps
- **Half-Holds with 3 Quick Flicks:** 20 reps

DAY TWENTY-EIGHT

- **Static Holds:** 25 seconds, 3 reps
- **Quick Flicks:** 20 reps
- **Elevator Exercises:** 10 reps
- **Half-Holds with 3 Quick Flicks:** 20 reps

DAY TWENTY-NINE

- **Static Holds:** 33 seconds, 1 rep (or keep working toward this goal)
- **Quick Flicks:** 20 reps
- **Elevator Exercises:** 10 reps
- **Half-Holds with 3 Quick Flicks:** 20 reps

DAY THIRTY: ASSESSMENT DAY

Check your strength by contracting your pelvic floor muscles. You should be able to:

- Feel your pelvic floor muscles lift toward your nose when you contract them

- Sustain your hold
- Show coordinated movement control in both the elevation and descent of your elevator exercises
- Perform quick contractions with control

Important Note: If you haven't quite reached the repetitions and durations listed on Day Twenty-Nine—don't worry! Continue with the exercises from Day Twenty-Nine (or wherever you're feeling comfortable in the program). Remember, it typically takes twelve weeks of consistent practice to see optimal results.

UNDERSTANDING BLADDER FUNCTION

Rebuilding your pelvic floor strength will require consistent effort and can take up to twelve weeks. However, if you are noticing new symptoms, it can be helpful to understand common pelvic floor issues, the key factors involved, and how your healthcare team can support you in addressing them.

The Four Factors of Continence

Bladder control relies on the following four key elements working together:

1. HORMONAL SUPPORT: Estrogen plays an important role in promoting blood flow to your urethra (the tube that connects your bladder to the outside). Your healthcare provider might prescribe topical estrogen to help support tissue health.

2. FASCIAL SUPPORT: The pelvic floor fascia support your bladder, uterus, and other organs. These connective tissues need time to recover and regain optimal function.

3. MUSCULAR FUNCTION: The pelvic floor muscles (and the nerves that supply them) support your pelvic organs and play a vital role in maintaining continence.

4. BLADDER HABITS: Your bladder function is influenced by its filling patterns and your daily routines.

COMMON PELVIC FLOOR ISSUES

Stress Incontinence

Stress incontinence occurs during activities that increase abdominal pressure, such as coughing, sneezing, running, or laughing. Think of it as a pressure competition: If your pelvic floor muscles and urethral closure mechanism can generate more pressure than the activity, you stay dry. If not, urinary leakage occurs.

Research shows that starting pelvic floor exercises at any point during the first year postpartum can help reduce urinary leakage. Aim to complete 40 to 50 pelvic floor exercises daily whenever possible. Remember, factors like the number of pregnancies you've had, your age, or your body weight don't determine success—pelvic floor training can work for many.

Urgency and Frequency

With or without leakage, if you're urinating frequently in small amounts or experiencing intense or painful urges to urinate, there may be a behavioral component to address. Your medical team will rule out other reasons, such as an infection, first.

These conditions can often be effectively managed with the help of a pelvic health specialist. In the meantime, here are some strategies to consider:

- Distribute your water intake evenly throughout the day.
- Monitor your hydration needs, and adjust as needed.
- Regulate your fluid intake based on your activity level, not time-based metrics.
- Limit bladder irritants, such as caffeine or acidic foods.
- Use distraction techniques to delay urination unless it's painful.
- Discuss the potential influence of estrogen with your healthcare provider.
- Make sure you're not constipated.
- Use the restroom frequently if you're experiencing painful, intense urges to pee.

Nighttime Urination

While it's normal to use the bathroom when you're awake for nighttime feedings, your bladder shouldn't be the reason you're waking up. If frequent nighttime urination is disrupting your sleep, bladder training—practicing to resist the urge to urinate when it's only a small amount—may help. Consult your pelvic health specialist or healthcare team for guidance on this process.

Understanding Prolapse

Prolapse occurs when pelvic organs shift from their normal position due to changes in the supporting structures. You might notice:

- Feelings of openness or bulging
- Pressure or heaviness
- Difficulty with bowel movements
- Low back pain
- Leakage after emptying your bladder or during intimacy

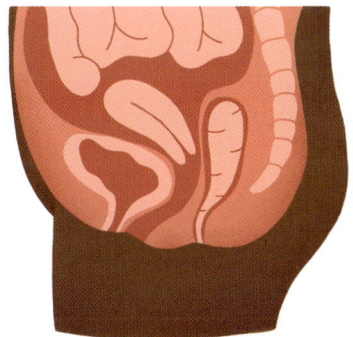

NORMAL

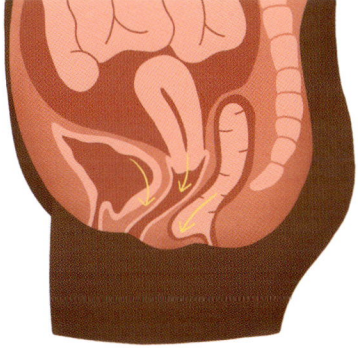

THREE TYPES OF PROLAPSE

The good news is that there are several support options available, including:

- Pelvic floor muscle training
- Pessaries
- Specialized pelvic health rehabilitation

MANAGING DAILY LIFE WITH INCONTINENCE

Building the strength needed to restore your continence takes time, but today's innovations for managing pelvic floor symptoms make it easier than ever to return to exercise postpartum and stay active for years to come. Options include:

- Absorbent workout underwear designed for movement
- Specialized athletic shorts with built-in support
- High-absorption pads for additional security

When returning to cardiovascular exercise postpartum, you might notice decreased pelvic floor tone after your workout, which can sometimes create a feeling of heaviness. While this is often normal, it's a good idea to discuss any concerns with your healthcare team. You might also try exercising at a different time of day and monitoring your symptoms to identify any patterns.

The Pessary: A Support Option for Recovery

After childbirth the ligaments and tissues supporting your pelvic organs may be more stretched than before, which can lead to concerns such as pelvic heaviness or incontinence. A pessary, which is a silicone device designed to provide support, can help manage these symptoms.

FROM THE PRO
Jessica's Perspective on Support

Think of a pessary like an ankle brace or eyeglasses—it's simply a tool to support your body while you need it. Many women find that using one during exercise gives them the confidence to return to the activities they love.

A pessary provides essential support for your pelvic organs. Many women learn to insert and remove it themselves and only use it during high-impact activities such as exercise, while others prefer to wear it throughout the day for consistent support. A pessary presses against the walls of the vagina and urethra and helps prevent leakage during high-pressure activities like jumping, running, or even laughing. Some types of pessaries can also provide support for the rectum and uterus.

Studies show remarkable success with pessary use, with more than 80 percent of women reporting improvement when using one consistently for a year or longer. As a cost-effective, non-surgical solution, a pessary might be worth discussing for issues with prolapse and urination. Consult your healthcare provider to determine if a pessary could benefit your recovery.

Pro tip: If you experience less leakage when using tampons during menstruation, a pessary might be particularly beneficial for you.

Note: Always wait for clearance from your healthcare provider, which you'll typically get at six to eight weeks postpartum, before inserting anything into your vagina. Your postpartum checkup is an excellent opportunity for your healthcare provider to assess pelvic floor strength, check for signs of prolapse, and evaluate how your incisions are healing.

RETURNING TO ACTIVITY: ASSESSING YOUR READINESS

The guidance on returning to activity when experiencing pelvic floor symptoms can often feel contradictory, but we're here to help.

MYTH: You must limit your activity if you have pelvic floor leakage.

Some people suggest returning to activity when you feel ready, while others strictly advise against any activity that causes leakage.

The reality lies somewhere in between. Specific strength markers, symptoms, and pelvic floor flexibility should guide your progress. Before advancing to more demanding activities, it's important to assess your pelvic floor function.

You can use the Self-Assessment Tool below to evaluate whether your body is ready to return to activity. Keep in mind that self-assessments are not a substitute for professional healthcare. Always consult your healthcare provider before beginning a new exercise program.

Self-Assessment Tools

VISUAL ASSESSMENT

Using a mirror, check for the following:

- A gaping, wide, or enlarged vagina opening
- Visible protrusions during a 6 to 8 second push, repeated three times (similar to having a bowel movement or pushing during labor)

If you notice any of the above, it's important to focus on strengthening your pelvic floor before returning to moderate or high-level exercise.

Note: Consult your medical provider if you have any signs of protrusion or gaping, as some movement is normal and some needs medical guidance.

MUSCLE FUNCTION

Pelvic floor strength is a vital part of postpartum pelvic health. When your pelvic floor muscles are strong enough, they will help guide your return to moderate and high-level exercise. To assess your pelvic floor strength, try the steps below.

During a pelvic floor contraction, check:

- If you feel the muscles lift toward your nose
- Whether the vagina and anus visibly close and lift with the urethra
- The quality of and control over the movement

Aftering drinking 3 cups of water or during your largest bathroom break of the day, have a watch or timer available and wait for a strong urge to pee. Then:

- Start peeing.
- Attempt to stop the flow of urine 5 seconds after initiating your stream.
- Monitor how long it takes to stop peeing and check if it takes less than 3 seconds.

Note: Do this test sparingly to reduce bladder infection risk as research is limited.

REVIEW

If your muscle function assessment yields positive results, this may indicate that your pelvic floor strength is sufficient for moderate and high-level exercise.

If you don't notice your pelvic floor muscles lifting or stopping the flow in less than 3 seconds, they may need further strengthening. This will help to prevent potential pelvic floor issues in the future, especially if your visual assessment shows gaping or protrusions.

Your Return-to-Activity Checklist

Before progressing to high-impact activities, assess your pelvic floor readiness with these key indicators:

- You have clearance from your health-care provider.
- You can perform ten Quick Flicks.
- You can hold 8 to 12 pelvic contractions for 6 to 8 seconds each.
- You can sustain a 33-second pelvic contraction at 50 percent of your strength.
- You don't experience leakage during daily activities. (This is not an absolute requirement but a sign that it may be time for a consultation.)
- You don't feel a sense of pressure in the pelvis.

While the assessment above offers general guidance, healthcare providers now rely on specific measurements to help determine when it's safe to return to high-level activity. They will assess if you meet one or both of the following:

- They will measure your pelvic floor opening from the urethra to the anal opening (called your GH and PB) to see if it's less than 7 centimeters.
- They will measure your pelvic floor strength rating to ensure it's at least 3 on a scale of 5.

Remember, these measurements serve as guidelines, not rigid rules. The key is working with your healthcare team to find what works best for your body to support your pelvic floor health and exercise.

LOOKING AHEAD

The pelvic floor rehabilitation work you've learned in this chapter forms the foundation for everything that follows. These exercises aren't just a temporary phase of recovery—they're lifelong tools that will continue to serve you as you regain strength and return to the activities you love.

In the next chapter, we'll guide you through a progressive twelve-week training program designed to systematically rebuild strength from your core outward. This comprehensive program builds upon the pelvic floor awareness and control you've developed here, expanding outward to restore full-body strength and function.

The beauty of this approach is that these exercises can all be done in tandem with your pelvic floor rehabilitation work. Rather than replacing what you've learned, the upcoming program enhances and supports your pelvic floor recovery while gradually reintroducing more complex movements and challenges.

Molly Huddle

2x Olympian, 28x US champion

My biggest concern around fitness during my first pregnancy was navigating the uncertainty of my new physical limits. As a professional distance runner with twenty-two years of training experience, I was accustomed to 70 to 90 miles per week with twice-daily sessions, but pregnancy required a completely different approach. How much should I slow down? How much volume should I reduce? In the end, I managed my anxieties about training too hard by doing less and running easier than I probably could have.

What surprised me most was discovering which elements of my training felt good versus what didn't work during pregnancy. I expected to enjoy slower activities like long runs and tempo workouts, thinking I'd gravitate toward the pool and yoga while avoiding the weight room and faster running. The reality was completely opposite—I actually enjoyed short, quicker reps and felt comfortable in the gym, but I dropped my long run from the schedule almost immediately. Swimming, yoga classes, and pool runs felt biomechanically awkward.

During my first trimester, I reduced my volume to about 60 percent of normal and slowed workouts to whatever felt manageable. By the second trimester, I was doing 40 to 50 percent of my normal training volume. The third trimester brought an even more conservative approach—mostly easy runs, easy cross-training, walking, drills, and strides, along with light strength work.

Around week 24, my daughter's in-utero arrhythmia was detected, which made me too nervous to push harder than an easy effort. One discovery that surprised me was how much better I felt on days when I managed to get even 20 minutes of movement. I experienced less nausea, reduced swelling, and improved mood. For cross-training, I really enjoyed the ElliptiGO and cycling—they felt like running but with just enough weight-bearing removed to be comfortable.

Postpartum brought its own surprises and challenges. Despite maintaining strength work throughout pregnancy, my muscular strength took longer to return than expected. My return-to-sport timeline began with light rehab exercises and scar work with Jessica around three weeks postpartum, following my cesarean delivery. I attempted my first run-walk intervals at eight weeks postpartum, had my first continuous 20-minute run just over ten weeks postpartum, and rejoined professional workouts around 16.5 weeks.

The most frustrating setback came at ten months postpartum when I developed a femoral stress fracture. Just as I'd returned to good shape, I lost more opportunities to qualify for events. I wish I'd known more about the relationship between breastfeeding and bone health, as my period didn't return until 14 months postpartum.

My advice to athletes wanting to stay active during pregnancy is to seek guidance from a physical therapist to avoid biomechanical injuries. The research around limits for pregnant athletes is sparse, which can be scary. I found comfort in speaking with other professional athlete mothers who had maintained significant training loads successfully.

For so long, my body performed in sports that I almost forgot it could do other amazing things. Pregnancy filled me with awe for my body's capabilities beyond athletics. Postpartum, I felt frustrated by the slow pace of returning to my former self while breastfeeding. I should have been more patient and understanding.

The biggest change as an athlete is that my career isn't the priority anymore. It's still high on my list and I love it, but it now fits around my family's schedule. My advice to other athlete mothers: do what you can handle athletically, and check that it still feels empowering and energizing in your new life. It's okay to step back for a while. There's time to return or explore movement that fits your new life better.

CHAPTER 19

Your Twelve-Week Core and Strength Training Program

PHASE ONE: FOUNDATION BUILDING (WEEKS ONE TO FOUR)

It takes your body about four weeks to coordinate muscle activity when starting a new exercise. Focus on refining your movement patterns by revisiting the techniques you learned in earlier chapters.

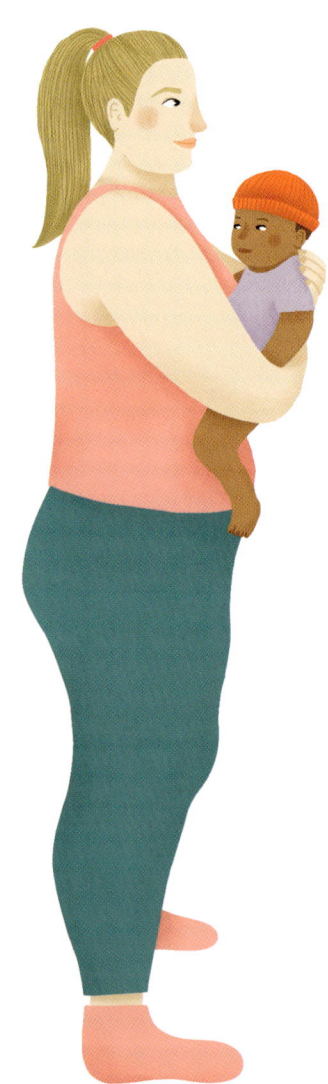

WEEK ONE: Reconnection

Days One and Two: Rest and celebrate bringing your baby into the world. Prioritize bonding, recovery, and basic self-care.

Days Three and Four: Start focusing on gently controlling your entire core as you move through your daily activities.

EXERCISE	FREQUENCY	PAGE
Core Engagement Holds	10 reps, 2 sets	215
Sit to Stand	10 reps, 2 sets	250

Days Five to Seven: First Exercise Series

EXERCISE	FREQUENCY	PAGE
Arm Lifts	10 reps per side, 2 sets	207
Heel Slides	10 reps per side, 2 sets	223
Knee Fall Outs	10 reps per side, 2 sets	224
Seated Pelvic Tilts on Ball	10 reps per side, 2 sets	238

Perform series 1–3 times daily

WEEK TWO: Building Patterns

Life with a newborn means being flexible. This week's three workouts introduce a structured program that targets different areas during each session. Try to schedule some time every day to complete a few exercises whenever possible. Remember, consistency is key. It's better to do a few exercises each day consistently than to sporadically complete them all at once.

Core Day

	EXERCISE	FREQUENCY	PAGE
CORE CONTROL	Knee Straighteners	10 reps per side, 2 sets	226
	Marches	10 reps per side, 2 sets	230
BREATHING AND MOBILITY WORK	Breathing	2-3 minutes	199
	Scalene Stretch	30 seconds per side, 1-2 sets	235
	Standing Snow Angels	10 reps, 1-2 sets	256

Upper Body Day

	EXERCISE	FREQUENCY	PAGE
STRENGTH SERIES	Rows (Banded)	10 reps, 1-2 sets	232
	Triceps (Banded)	10 reps, 1-2 sets	257
	Front Arm Raises (Weighted)	10 reps, 1-2 sets	220
	Pull Downs (Banded)	10 reps, 1-2 sets	232
MOBILITY WORK	Child's Pose Stretch	30 seconds per position, 1–2 sets	214
	Seated Twist Stretch	30 seconds per side, 1-2 sets	239

Lower Body Day

	EXERCISE	FREQUENCY	PAGE
HIP AND KNEE SERIES	Seated Hip Abduction	10 reps, 1–2 sets	236
	Seated Leg Extensions (Banded)	10 reps per side, 1–2 sets	237
	Seated Leg Curls (Banded)	10 reps per side, 1–2 sets	237
FOOT AND ANKLE SERIES	Four-Way Ankle (Banded)	10 reps in each direction per side, 1-2 sets	220
	Arch Lifts	20 reps, 1–2 sets	207

WEEK THREE: Increasing Complexity

Core Day

	EXERCISE	FREQUENCY	PAGE
CORE CONTROL	Core Curl Ups	10 reps, 1–2 sets	214
	Arm Lifts (Weighted)	10 reps per side, 2 sets	208
	Leg Lifts	10 reps per side, 2 sets	228
	Marches	10 reps per side, 2 sets	230
MOBILITY WORK	Breathing	2–3 minutes	199
	Scalene Stretch	30 seconds per side, 1–2 sets	235
	Standing Snow Angels	10 reps, 1–2 sets	256

Upper Body Day

	EXERCISE	FREQUENCY	PAGE
STRENGTH SERIES	Triceps (Banded)	10 reps, 1–2 sets	257
	Front Arm Raises (Weighted)	10 reps, 1–2 sets	220
	Pull Downs (Banded)	10 reps, 1–2 sets	232
MOBILITY WORK	Child's Pose Stretch	30 seconds per position, 1–2 sets	214
	Seated Twist Stretch	30 seconds per side, 1–2 sets	239

WELLNESS INSIGHT
Research shows that dedicated pelvic floor muscle training leads to complete symptom resolution in ⅓ to ½ of women, while nearly 3 out of 4 experience significant improvement. These odds increase when working with a professional, instead of training on your own, make you eight times more likely to succeed.

Lower Body Day

	EXERCISE	FREQUENCY	PAGE
HIP AND KNEE SERIES	Seated Hip Abduction (Banded)	10 reps, 1–2 sets	236
	Seated Hip Adduction	10 reps, 1–2 sets	236
	Seated Leg Extensions (Banded)	10 reps per side, 1–2 sets	237
	Seated Leg Curls (Banded)	10 reps per side, 1–2 sets	237
FOOT AND ANKLE SERIES	Four-Way Ankle (Banded)	10 reps in each direction per side, 1–2 sets	220
	Arch Lifts	20 reps, 1–2 sets	207

WEEK FOUR: Building Intensity

WELLNESS INSIGHT
Here's an encouraging milestone to work toward: When you can maintain a gentle pelvic floor contraction at about half of your maximum strength for 33 seconds, you're much more likely to stay dry during daily activities.

Core Day

	EXERCISE	FREQUENCY	PAGE
CORE CONTROL	Core Curl Ups	10 reps, 1–2 sets	214
	Arm Lifts (Weighted)	10 reps per side, 2 sets	208
	Four Point Arm Lifts	10 reps per side, 2 sets	219
MOBILITY WORK	Breathing	2–3 minutes	199
	Scalene Stretch	30 seconds per side, 1–2 sets	235
	Standing Snow Angels	10 reps, 1–2 sets	256

Upper Body Day

	EXERCISE	FREQUENCY	PAGE
STRENGTH SERIES	Rows (Banded)	10 reps, 1–2 sets	232
	Triceps (Banded)	10 reps, 1–2 sets	257
	Seated Shoulder Press (Weighted)	10 reps, 1–2 sets	239
	Pull Downs (Banded)	10 reps, 1–2 sets	232
MOBILITY WORK	Child's Pose Stretch	30 seconds per position, 1–2 sets	214
	Seated Twist Stretch	30 seconds per side, 1-2 sets	239

Lower Body Day

	EXERCISE	FREQUENCY	PAGE
HIP AND KNEE SERIES	Seated Hip Abduction (Banded)	10 reps, 1–2 sets	236
	Seated Hip Adduction	10 reps, 1–2 sets	236
	Seated Leg Extensions (Banded)	10 reps per side, 1–2 sets	237
	Seated Leg Curls (Banded)	10 reps per side, 1–2 sets	237
FOOT AND ANKLE SERIES	Four-Way Ankle (Banded)	10 reps in each direction per side, 1–2 sets	220
	Arch Lifts	20 reps, 1–2 sets	207

PHASE TWO: PROGRESSIVE LOADING (WEEKS FIVE AND SIX)

WELLNESS INSIGHT As you think about returning to exercise, take some time to envision your six-month and one-year fitness goals. Having these longer-term goals in mind can help you pace yourself appropriately, allowing your body the time it needs to heal while staying focused on your ultimate vision. Remember, a thoughtful approach to fitness progression now leads to sustainable strength later.

After four weeks of muscle activation work, your body is ready to start building strength in your core, arms, and legs—empowering you to care for your baby and return to the activities you love. During this phase we'll also focus on your upper back mobility to help it recover from hours spent holding and nursing your baby.

PROGRESSION NOTE

Each exercise builds on the previous week. Progress only when you:

• Can complete your current exercises with proper form
• Are able to control your breathing
• Feel in control during movements
• Don't experience any pain

Start with lighter resistance (weights or bands) and gradually increase it while maintaining good technique.

WEEK FIVE: Gaining Strength

Core Day

	EXERCISE	FREQUENCY	PAGE
CORE CONTROL	Core Curl Ups	10 reps, 1–2 sets	214
	Four Point Leg Lifts	10 reps per side, 2 sets	219
MOBILITY WORK	Foam Roller Upper Back Stretch	1–2 sets	218
	Standing Snow Angels	10 reps, 1–2 sets	256

Upper Body Day

	EXERCISE	FREQUENCY	PAGE
STRENGTH SERIES	Split-Stance Row (Banded)	10 reps per side, 1–2 sets	252
	Front Arm Raises (Weighted)	10 reps, 1–2 sets	220
	Diagonal Pulls (Banded)	10 reps per side, 1–2 sets	216
	Wall Push-Up Plus	10 reps, 1–2 sets	258
MOBILITY WORK	Side-Lying Rotation Stretch	30 seconds per side, 1–2 sets	241
	Thread Needle Stretch	30 seconds per side, 1–2 sets	257
	Counter Stretch	30 seconds per position, 1–2 sets	215

Lower Body Day

	EXERCISE	FREQUENCY	PAGE
HIP AND KNEE SERIES	Standing Hip Abduction	10 reps per side, 1–2 sets	252
	Standing Hip Adduction	10 reps per side, 1–2 sets	253
	Seated Marches	10 reps per side, 1–2 sets	237
MOBILITY WORK	Dynamic Adductor Stretch	10–15 reps per movement, per side, 1-2 sets	217
	Standing Hip Flexor Stretch	30 seconds per side, 1–2 sets	254

WEEK SIX: Building Intensity

Core Day

	EXERCISE	FREQUENCY	PAGE
CORE CONTROL	Core Curl Ups	10 reps, 1–2 sets	214
	Four Point Opposite Arm and Leg Lifts	10 reps per side, 2 sets	219
MOBILITY WORK	Foam Roller Upper-Back Stretch	1-2 sets	218
	Standing Snow Angels	10 reps, 1–2 sets	256

Upper Body Day

	EXERCISE	FREQUENCY	PAGE
STRENGTH SERIES	Split-Stance Row (Banded)	10 reps per side, 1–2 sets	252
	Front Arm Raises (Weighted)	10 reps, 1–2 sets	220
	Diagonal Pulls (Banded)	10 reps per side, 1–2 sets	216
	Wall Push-Up Plus	10 reps, 1–2 sets	258
MOBILITY WORK	Side-Lying Rotation Stretch	30 seconds per side, 1–2 sets	241
	Thread Needle Stretch	30 seconds per side, 1–2 sets	257
	Counter Stretch	30 seconds per position, 1–2 sets	215

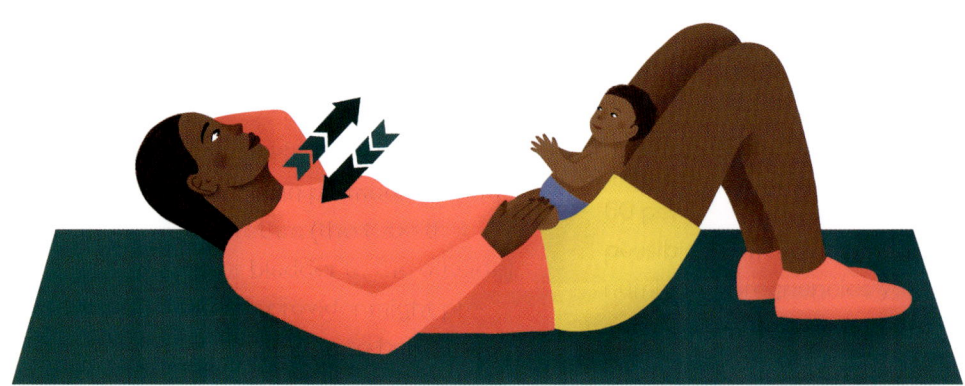

CORE CURL UPS

Lower Body Day

	EXERCISE	FREQUENCY	PAGE
HIP AND KNEE SERIES	Standing Hip Abduction (Banded)	10 reps per side, 1–2 sets	252
	Seated Marches (Banded)	10 reps per side, 1–2 sets	238
	Mini Squats	10 reps, 1–2 sets	230
	Forward Lunges	10 reps per side, 1–2 sets	218
MOBILITY WORK	Dynamic Adductor Stretch	10–15 reps per movement, per side, 1-2 sets	217
	Standing Hip Flexor Stretch	30 seconds per side, 1–2 sets	254

PHASE THREE: FUNCTIONAL INTEGRATION (WEEKS SEVEN TO NINE)

Motherhood requires new ways of moving and lifting, so we've designed this phase to help you build the strength needed for all your daily movements as you care for your little one.

NOTE ON INTEGRATING BABY MOVEMENTS

- Use your baby's weight as natural resistance when appropriate.
- Ensure that you're holding your baby securely during all movements.
- Start with basic holds before adding movement.
- Always prioritize your baby's safety and comfort.

WEEK SEVEN: Integrating Daily Movements

Core Day

	EXERCISE	FREQUENCY	PAGE
CORE CONTROL	Core Curl Ups (Banded)	10 reps, 1–2 sets	215
	Bridges	10 reps, 1-2 sets	212
	Medium Squats with Baby	10 reps, 1-2 sets	230
	Forward Lunges with Baby	10 reps per side, 1–2 sets	218
MOBILITY WORK	Foam Roller Upper Back Stretch	1-2 sets	218
	Standing Snow Angels	10 reps, 1-2 sets	256

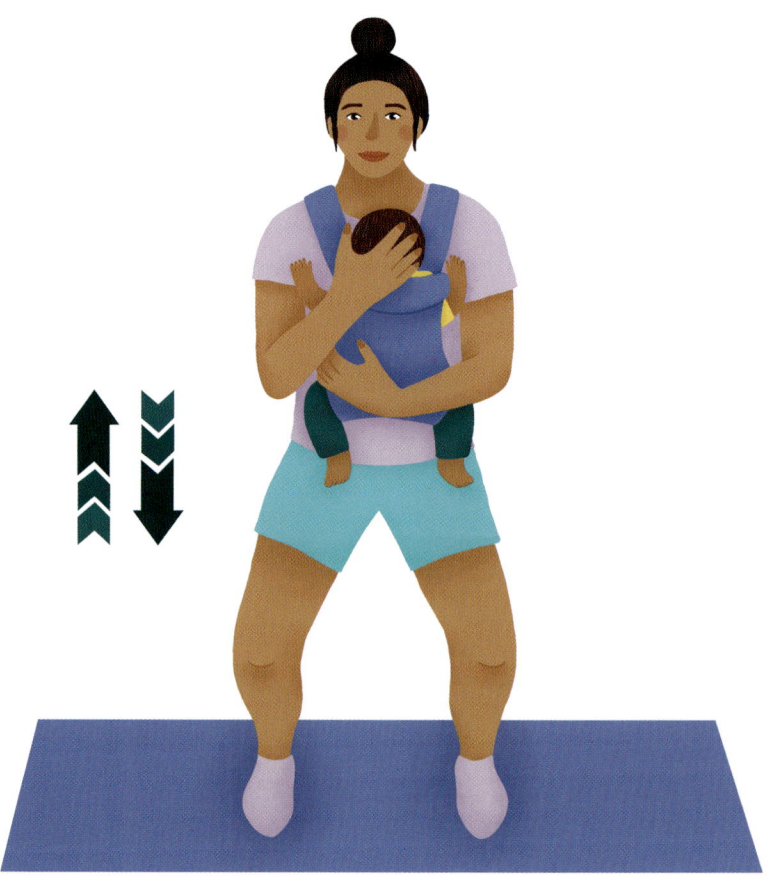

MEDIUM SQUATS WITH BABY

Upper Body Day

	EXERCISE	FREQUENCY	PAGE
STRENGTH SERIES	Split-Stance Row (Banded)	10 reps per side, 1–2 sets	252
	Front Arm Raises (Weighted)	10 reps, 1–2 sets	220
	Diagonal Pulls (Banded)	10 reps per side, 1–2 sets	216
	Wall Push-Up Plus	10 reps, 1–2 sets	258
MOBILITY WORK	Side-LyingRotation Stretch	30 seconds per side, 1–2 sets	241
	Thread Needle Stretch	30 seconds per side, 1–2 sets	257
	Counter Stretch	30 seconds per position, 1–2 sets	215

Lower Body Day

	EXERCISE	FREQUENCY	PAGE
HIP AND KNEE SERIES	Side Lunges	10 reps per side, 1–2 sets	242
	Medium Squats with Baby	10 reps, 1–2 sets	230
	Side-Lying Hip Abduction with Baby	10 reps per side, 1–2 sets	240
	Side-Lying Clamshells with Baby	10 reps per side, 1–2 sets	239
	Single-Leg Balance	2 reps per side, 1–2 sets	245
MOBILITY WORK	Dynamic Adductor Stretch	10–15 reps per movement, per side, 1–2 sets	217
	Standing Hip Flexor Stretch	30 seconds per side, 1–2 sets	254

WELLNESS INSIGHT
If you're planning to run with a stroller, wait until your baby has strong neck control and can sit independently, which typically happens when they're around six to nine months old. Start with easy runs that allow you to pause if needed to tend to your baby. Keep in mind that running with a stroller requires more energy and affects your form, so adjust your expectations and enjoy this new way of sharing movement with your little one.

WEEK EIGHT: Building Intensity

For this phase, we've combined two core and hip days to help you succeed in returning to high-level activities. Lifting your baby will continue to engage your upper body, but if you find the previous upper body strengthening exercises valuable, feel free to keep incorporating them.

Day One

	EXERCISE	FREQUENCY	PAGE
CORE AND LEG SERIES	Bear Plank Knee Taps	10 reps per side, 1–2 sets	208
	Bridges with Heel Lifts	10 reps per side, 1–2 sets	213
	Full Squats	10 reps, 1–2 sets	230
	Front Step Downs	10 reps per side, 1–2 sets	221
	Side Step Downs	10 reps per side, 1–2 sets	244
	Kneeling Side Plank	2 sets per side	227
	Calf Raises	10 reps, 1–2 sets	213
MOBILITY WORK	Standing Quadricep Stretch	30 seconds per side, 1–2 sets	255

PROGRESSION NOTE

Use these indicators to evaluate if you're ready to progress:

- Exercises feel challenging but achievable.
- You don't experience any pain during or after movements.
- You're able to control your breathing.
- Your core engagement is consistent.
- Daily activities feel stable.

Day Two

	EXERCISE	FREQUENCY	PAGE
CORE AND LEG SERIES	Core Curl Ups (Banded)	10 reps, 1–2 sets	215
	Glute Wall Reach	10 reps per side, 1–2 sets	222
	Side-Lying Hip Abduction (Banded)	10 reps per side, 1–2 sets	240
	Single-Leg Balance Clock Reaches	5 reps per side, 1–2 sets	245
	Side-Lying Clamshells (Banded)	10 reps per side, 1–2 sets	240
	Kneeling Pallof Press (Banded)	10 reps per side, 1–2 sets	226
	Bent-Knee Calf Raises	20 reps, 1–2 sets	210
MOBILITY WORK	Calf Stretch	30 seconds per side, 1–2 sets	213
	Bent-Knee Calf Stretch	30 seconds per side, 1–2 sets	211

Day Three: Pick Your Favorites

Select 3–5 of the most effective exercises from your previous workouts.

WEEK NINE: Functional Progression

Day One

	EXERCISE	FREQUENCY	PAGE
CORE AND LEG SERIES	Bear Plank Leg Lifts	10 reps per side, 1–2 sets	209
	70/30 Bridges	10 reps per side, 1–2 sets	206
	70/30 Squats	10 reps per side, 1–2 sets	207
	Front Step Downs	10 reps per side, 1–2 sets	221
	Side Step Downs	10 reps per side, 1–2 sets	244
	Side Plank Leg Lifts (Kneeling)	10 reps per side, 1–2 sets	243
	70/30 Calf Raises	10 reps per side, 1–2 sets	206
MOBILITY WORK	Standing Quadricep Stretch	30 seconds per side, 1–2 sets	255

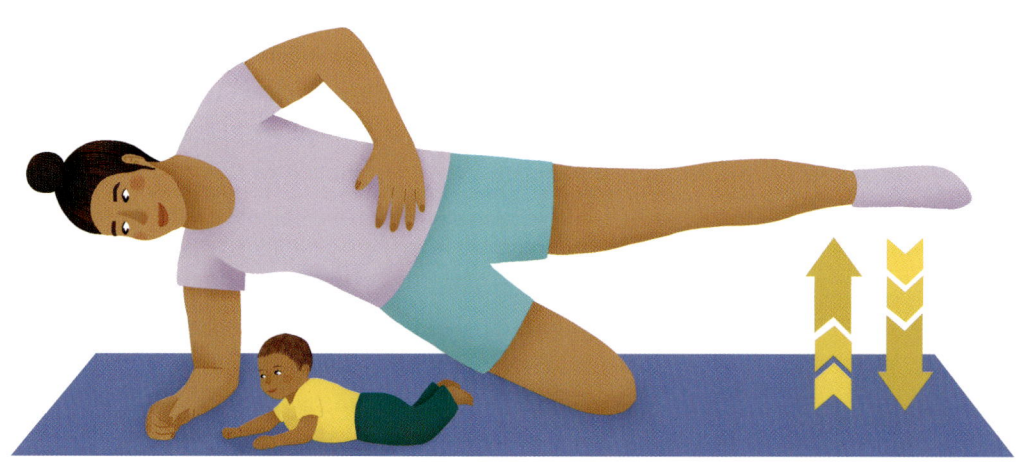

SIDE PLANK LEG LIFTS (KNEELING)

Day Two

	EXERCISE	FREQUENCY	PAGE
CORE AND LEG SERIES	Core Curl Ups (Banded)	10 reps, 1–2 sets	215
	Side Step Downs	10 reps per side, 1–2 sets	244
	Runner's Balance Challenges	10 reps per side, 1–2 sets	232
	Side Steps	10 reps each direction, 1–2 sets	244
	Single-Leg Balance Clock Reaches	5 reps per side, 1–2 sets	245
	Kneeling Side Plank Clamshells	10 reps per side, 1–2 sets	227
	Single-Leg to Single-Arm Row (Banded)	10 reps per side, 1–2 sets	250
	Bent-Knee 70/30 Calf Raises	20 reps per side, 1–2 sets	210
MOBILITY WORK	Calf Stretch	30 seconds per side, 1–2 sets	213
	Bent-Knee Calf Stretch	30 seconds per side, 1–2	211

Day Three

	EXERCISE	FREQUENCY	PAGE
HIP STRENGTH	Standing Hip Adduction (Banded)	10 reps per side, 1–2 sets	253
PLYOMETRICS	Jump Prep	8 reps, 2 sets	224
	Hops (Banded)	8 reps, 2 sets	224

PICK YOUR FAVORITES

Select 3-5 of the most effective exercises from your previous workouts to round out your Day Three exercises.

PHASE FOUR: ATHLETIC PREPARATION (WEEKS TEN TO TWELVE)

As we move into athletic preparation, many of the movements required for higher-level activities rely heavily on hip, leg, and core strength. Mastering these exercises will help set you up for success when you assess your readiness to return to high-intensity activities. If the exercises become too challenging to progress, it's okay to stay at a level where you can maintain proper form. Adjust your timeline as needed to ensure steady, safe progress.

WEEK TEN: Advanced Integration

WELLNESS INSIGHT
If running while nursing feels right for you, trust that choice. Your milk supply and quality will remain intact, and your baby will continue to develop normally. The bonus? Your self-care supports both you and your baby's well-being, and you'll be modeling the importance of taking care of your own health and wellness needs to your little one.

Day One

	EXERCISE	FREQUENCY	PAGE
CORE AND LEG SERIES	Core Curl Ups (Banded)	10 reps, 1–2 sets	215
	Bear Plank Leg Lifts	10 reps per side, 1–2 sets	209
	70/30 Bridges	10 reps per side, 1–2 sets	206
	Single-Leg Squats at Wall	10 reps per side, 1–2 sets	248
	Front Step Downs	10 reps per side, 1–2 sets	221
	Side Plank Leg Lifts (Kneeling)	10 reps per side, 1–2 sets	243
	Single-Leg Calf Raises	10 reps per side, 1–2 sets	247
MOBILITY WORK	Standing Quadricep Stretch	30 seconds per side, 1–2 sets	255

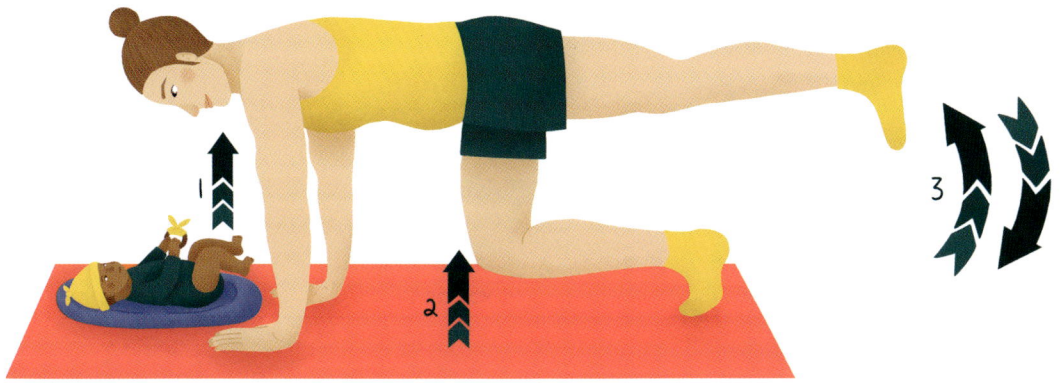

BEAR PLANK LEG LIFTS

Day Two

	EXERCISE	FREQUENCY	PAGE
CORE AND LEG SERIES	Low Bicycle	10 reps per side, 1–2 sets	229
	Side Step Downs	10 reps per side, 1–2 sets	244
	Runner's Balance Challenges	10 reps per side, 1–2 sets	232
	Side Steps (Banded)	10 reps each direction, 1–2 sets	244
	Single-Leg Balance Clock Reaches	5 reps per side, 1–2 sets	245
	Kneeling Side Plank Clamshells	10 reps per side, 1–2 sets	227
	Single-Leg to Single-Arm Row (Banded)	10 reps per side, 1–2 sets	250
	Kneeling Side Plank Hip Drops	10 reps per side, 1–2 sets	227
	Bent-Knee Single-Leg Calf Raises	20 reps per side, 1–2 sets	211
MOBILITY WORK	Calf Stretch	30 seconds per side, 1–2 sets	213
	Bent-Knee Calf Stretch	30 seconds per side, 1–2 sets	211

Day Three

	EXERCISE	FREQUENCY	PAGE
HIP STRENGTH	Standing Hip Adduction (Banded)	10 reps per side, 1–2 sets	253
PLYOMETRICS	Double-Leg Hops (Forward/Backward)	8 reps, 2 sets	216
	Double-Leg Hops (Side-to-Side)	8 reps, 2 sets	217
	Ladder In/Outs	8 reps, 2 sets	228

Pick Your Favorites

Select 3–5 of the most effective exercises from your previous workouts.

STARTING PLYOMETRICS

Begin your plyometric training with double-leg movements, focusing on soft, quiet landings—just like a cat landing gracefully. Start with two sets of eight repetitions, resting 30–60 seconds between sets. This phase is about building quality movement patterns, not endurance. Master double-leg control before progressing to single-leg work, and allow your body to gradually adapt to higher-intensity training. The goal is to maintain 60 plyometric repetitions per week over the next 6–8 weeks.

WEEK ELEVEN: Building Intensity

Day One

	EXERCISE	FREQUENCY	PAGE
CORE AND LEG SERIES	Core Curl Ups (Banded)	10 reps, 1–2 sets	215
	Full Plank	2 sets per side	221
	Single-Leg Bridges	10 reps per side, 1–2 sets	246
	Single-Leg Squats	10 reps per side, 1–2 sets	248
	Front Step Downs	10 reps per side, 1–2 sets	221
	Side Plank	2 sets per side	243
	Single-Leg Calf Raises	10 reps per side, 1–2 sets	247
MOBILITY WORK	Standing Quadricep Stretch	30 seconds per side, 1–2 sets	255

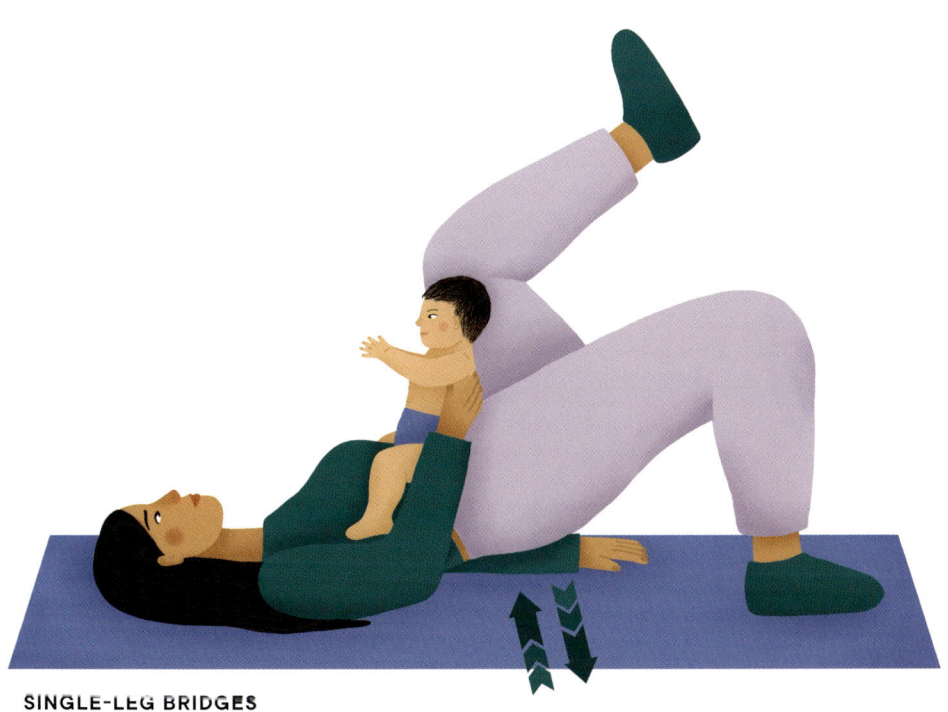

SINGLE-LEG BRIDGES

Day Two

	EXERCISE	FREQUENCY	PAGE
CORE AND LEG SERIES	Toe Taps	10 reps per side, 1–2 sets	257
	Side Step Downs	10 reps per side, 1–2 sets	244
	Split-Stance Romanian Deadlifts	10 reps per side, 1–2 sets	251
	Runner's Clamshells	10 reps per side, 1–2 sets	234
	Kneeling Side Plank Hip Drops with Leg Lift	10 reps per side, 1–2 sets	228
	Runner's Bent-Knee Calf Raises	20 reps per side, 1–2 sets	233
MOBILITY WORK	Calf Stretch	30 seconds per side, 1–2 sets	213
	Bent-Knee Calf Stretch	30 seconds per side, 1–2 sets	211

Day Three

	EXERCISE	FREQUENCY	PAGE
HIP STRENGTH	Wall Copenhagen with Runner's Drive	10 reps per side, 1–2 sets	258
PLYOMETRICS	Single-Leg Hops (Forward/Backward)	8 reps, 2 sets	247
	Single-Leg Hops (Side-to-Side)	8 reps, 2 sets	247
	Ladder In/Outs	8 reps, 2 sets	228

PICK YOUR FAVORITES

Select 3-5 of the most effective exercises from your previous workouts to round out your Day Three exercises.

WEEK TWELVE: Peak Performance

This week's exercises are designed to enhance your control over your body during athletic movements. While some exercises may progress faster than others, this is the time to nourish and flourish. Pay attention to the movements that come easily and those that may benefit from modifications. Sometimes, spending another one or two weeks at an easier level will help you safely progress while maintaining proper form and technique. Remember, progress isn't linear; consistency is what builds the foundation for lifelong wellness.

Day One

	EXERCISE	FREQUENCY	PAGE
CORE AND LEG SERIES	Full Plank	30 seconds, 1–2 sets	221
	Single-Leg Bridges (Weighted)	10 reps per side, 1–2 sets	246
	Single-Leg Squats to Runner's Drive	10 reps per side, 1–2 sets	248
	Front Step Downs	10 reps per side, 1–2 sets	221
	Side Plank Leg Lifts	10 reps per side, 1–2 sets	243
	Single-Leg Calf Raises (Weighted)	10 reps per side, 1–2 sets	247
MOBILITY WORK	Standing Quadricep Stretch	30 seconds per side, 1–2 sets	255

WELLNESS INSIGHT
If you're still experiencing urinary leakage, now is the time to consult your healthcare provider about additional options. The progress you've made over the last twelve weeks will likely plateau, and formal treatment for urinary leakage can help you improve further.

Day Two

	EXERCISE	FREQUENCY	PAGE
CORE AND LEG SERIES	Runner's Toe Taps	10 reps per side, 1–2 sets	235
	Split-Stance Romanian Deadlifts	10 reps per side, 1–2 sets	251
	Hip Thrusters	10 reps, 1–2 sets	223
	Runner's Clamshells (Banded)	10 reps per side, 1–2 sets	234
	Side Plank Hip Drops	10 reps per side, 1–2 sets	243
	Runner's Bent-Knee Calf Raises (Weighted)	20 reps per side, 1–2 sets	233
MOBILITY WORK	Calf Stretch	30 seconds per side, 1–2 sets	213
	Bent-Knee Calf Stretch	30 seconds per side, 1–2 sets	211

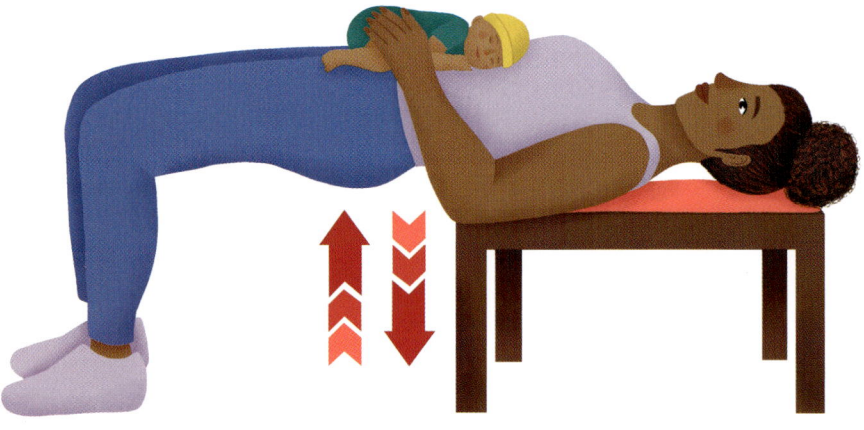

HIP THRUSTERS

Day Three

	EXERCISE	FREQUENCY	PAGE
HIP STRENGTH	Modified Copenhagen on Jump Box	1-2 sets per side	231
PLYOMETRICS	Scissor Jumps	8 reps, 2 sets	235
	Box Jumps	8 reps, 2 sets	211
	Box Taps	8 reps per side, 2 sets	212

PICK YOUR FAVORITES

Select 3 to 5 of the most effective exercises from your previous workouts to round out your Day Three exercises.

Week Twelve marks the start of continuous strength development, not the end. As you move forward, use the foundation you've established and gradually increase intensity while maintaining your form. Let your energy levels guide your training intensity, and keep engaging your core with the patterns you've learned. Consistent, mindful progression is more effective for building lasting strength than sporadic intense efforts.

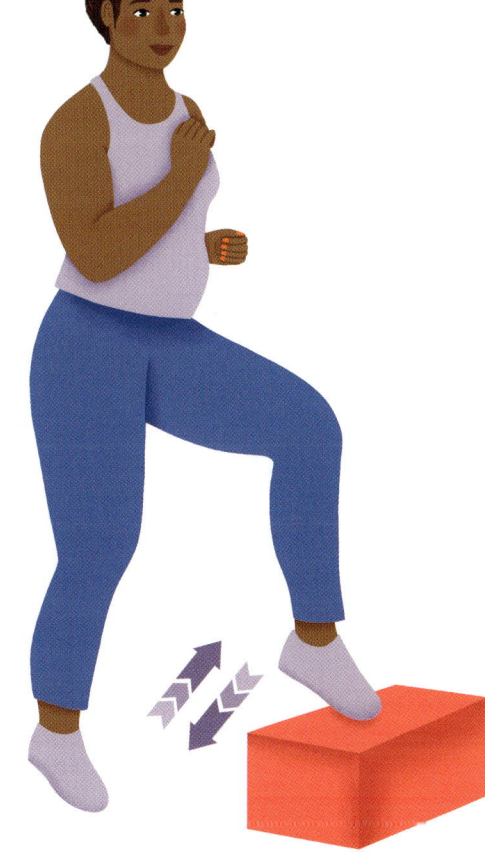

BOX TAPS

CHAPTER 20

Your Cardio Comeback

In addition to building core and hip strength, you might be eager to get back to more dynamic activities such as running, high-impact exercise, or intensive training. However, your return to cardiovascular fitness, much like your core recovery, will require a careful approach that allows for gradual progression.

THE TRUTH ABOUT RETURNING TO ACTIVITY

MYTH: You should return to high-level activities when you feel ready

While "When can I return to running, lifting, or CrossFit?" is perhaps the most common question in postpartum fitness, the answer isn't as simple as "when you feel ready." General guidelines suggest returning to high-level activities six to twelve weeks postpartum, but this time-line alone doesn't guarantee success.

A successful return to high-level activity involves considering multiple factors, including:

- Mental health readiness
- Physical healing status
- Previous training experience
- Relationship with exercise
- Current core and hip strength
- Rest and recovery capacity
- Nutritional support
- Current exercise tolerance

YOUR RETURN TO ACTIVITY JOURNEY

This program can be started at any stage of your postpartum journey. When combined with the Core and Strength Training Program from the previous chapter, you'll increase your chances of returning to activity safely and successfully.

Your Complete Strong as a Mother Program Checklist

- Follow the Twelve-Week *Strong as a Mother* Activity Progression.
- Continue the Core and Strength Training Program.
- On Day Thirty, assess your readiness with the Pelvic Floor Self-Assessment Tool on pages 153-154.
- On Week Twelve, complete the *Strong as a Mother* Assessment Protocol on pages 187-188.
- Choose appropriate activities.
- Follow foundational key concepts, such as our Guidelines for a Safe Return on page 189.

FROM THE PRO
Jessica's Assessment Insight

The most successful returns to activity come from respecting early checkpoints. They're not obstacles to overcome, but signposts that ensure you're on the right path.

Your Twelve-Week Strong as a Mother Activity Progression

This program respects your body's healing process while gradually and systematically increasing activity. Remember, you can start at any point postpartum—whenever it feels right for you. It's never too late to begin. If you're starting later than immediately postpartum, begin at Week Two.

Week One: Rest and Celebrate

Focus on rest, recovery, and celebrating your body's incredible achievement. Basic self-care like showering becomes your primary activity.

Week Two: First Steps Outside

Aim to go outside two or three times this week. This might mean simply sitting outside or going out to grab a coffee. Be sure to keep your walks short and to stay close to home by doing circles rather than a point to point walk.

Week Three: Building Consistency

Go outside three times this week.

- Walk at a manageable pace.
- Focus on duration; intensity will come later.
- Pay attention to your body's signals.

Week Four: Increasing Frequency

Aim to briefly go outside five times.

- Keep your walks short and stay close to home.
- Add one or two days of low-impact cardio, such as using a stationary bike, elliptical, or rowing machine (optional).
- Maintain a pace at which you can easily hold a conversation.

Week Five: Building Duration

Walk one mile or engage in an equivalent low-impact activity (five or six days).

- Focus on completing the distance comfortably.
- Increase the duration gradually before adding intensity.
- Listen to your body's feedback during each session.

Week Six: Adding Distance

Progress to two-mile walks (five or six days).

- Consider adding gentle uphill slopes for variety.
- Include power walking segments (optional).
- Maintain a pace at which you can hold a conversation throughout.

Week Seven: Increasing Endurance

Build up to three-mile walks (five or six days)

- Keep your pace comfortable but purposeful.
- Focus on maintaining good posture.
- Notice how your body responds to longer distances.

Week Eight: Reaching Milestones

Progress to four-mile walks at a brisk pace.

- Go swimming if you're fully healed (optional).
- Pay attention to your energy levels.
- Notice how your body recovers between sessions.

Week Nine: Introduction to Impact

- Jog, bike, or use a cardio exercise machine twice a week.
- Start with 5 minutes of up-tempo exercise.
- Progress to 10 minutes as comfortable.

- Use interval patterns, such as:
  - Alternate 1 minute of running with 5 minutes of walking (5 reps)
  - Alternate running and walking at equal length intervals in a 1-2-1-2-1-2-minute progression.
- Start incorporating dynamic warm-up exercises, such as high knees, figure-four walks, tin soldiers, A-skips and B-skips, side shuffles, toe/heel walks, and lunges with reach and rotation.

Week Ten: Reintroduction to Running

- Days One and Three: Alternate 1 minute of running with 1 minute of walking (7 reps).
- Day Six: Alternate 2 to 3 minutes of running with 1 minute of walking (5 reps).
- Keep working on your form.

Week Eleven: Building Running Base

- Day One: Alternate 2 to 3 minutes of running with 1 minute of walking (5 reps).
- Days Two and Three: Alternate 3 to 5 minutes of running with 1 minute of walking for a total of 20 minutes.
- Complete the *Strong as a Mother* Assessment Protocol on pages 187-188.
- Keep working on your form.

Week Twelve: Strengthening Running Base

- Continue to slowly build up to 30 minutes of running every other day as your ability allows.
- Take breaks to walk as needed.
- Focus on volume before intensity.
- Consider working with a running coach.
- Follow the Fundamental Rules on page 189.

A Professional's Perspective: The Reality of Returning to Exercise

Even elite athletes must approach postpartum running with patience and flexibility. Shannon's experience with her first postpartum run illustrates the physical and emotional challenges of this transition.

FROM THE PRO
Shannon's First Postpartum Run

I'll never forget my first postpartum run. It was August 30, 2018—two months to the day after I gave birth. I didn't want to start running, but I had to. Running was my job and, at that time, my sport did not offer maternity protection. Technically, I had already done my first race: I walked 5K at four weeks post-partum, carrying my daughter on my chest. It was necessary, but definitely not ideal: I had to protect my contract from being reduced or terminated. Two months postpartum my coach decided that it was time to start running again because I needed to prepare to race against the nation's best at Cross-Country Nationals—just six months after giving birth.

Jess, who had been my guide and my salvation throughout my pregnancy journey, came down to San Francisco to join me on my first run. I think she knew it would be difficult and she wanted to be there to provide moral support. She has a thorough "return to running" protocol, which we included in this book, and before I took my first running step, she made sure that I met all the milestones on her checklist.

Once I was cleared to run, we headed out. We decided to do my first run in San Francisco's Golden Gate Park—the same place I did my first run twenty years before as a high school freshman. It felt symbolically fitting to have my first run as a mom take place there too.

Together we drove to the Polo Fields, a 1200-meter dirt loop that had started as a home for horses but had become my go-to spot for a flat, soft surface run. I was anxious. It was all happening so fast. I was still tired and, if I'm being honest, a little resentful that I had to push my body so soon after my daughter's birth.

With Jess there, it felt a little less daunting. It's impossible not to feel positive in Jess's presence. Sensing my nerves, she kept the conversation light, distracting me from the swirl of thoughts racing through my head.

We hopped out of the car. I swung my arms and legs, partly to limber up my body and partly to hide how nervous I was.

As I stood there, delaying the inevitable, Jess asked my plan for my first run.

"How much are you thinking?" she asked.

"Twenty minutes," I said, thinking that seemed easy enough.

I saw the faintest smile creep across Jess's face, but she just nodded her head. "OK," she said. "Let's see how it goes."

We started jogging, and within three minutes, I was breathing heavily. My body felt sluggish, and my legs felt like lead.

"How do you feel?" Jess asked.

"Terrible," I replied. There was no sense in playing it cool. My struggle was obvious.

Jess laughed. "I thought twenty minutes might be a little much to start, but I wanted you to feel it out."

"Yeah . . ." I said, feeling defeated. But before I could melt into a puddle, Jess offered a solution.

"How about this: Why don't we jog for five minutes, then walk a little before running again? We'll turn this into a fartlek run. Your body just needs some time to get used to running again."

I felt my anxiety ease. Jess gave me permission to listen to my body and feel out this first run. Just like that, she'd shifted this overwhelming situation into a battle I could win.

"Sounds good," I blurted, feeling relieved.

We ran for five minutes, then walked for a minute. I took some deep breaths and chose to laugh rather than cry before we got going again. I ran a total of seventeen minutes, mostly in two-minute segments with one-minute walks in between.

I had a long way to go to reach world-class fitness, but that run, on that day, felt like a victory.

Learning from Experience

Shannon's story illustrates several important aspects of returning to running postpartum. Even as an Olympic athlete, she had to:

- Start more gradually than expected
- Modify her plans in the moment
- Accept support and guidance
- Listen to her body's signals
- Celebrate small victories

While most of us won't face the pressure of professional contracts, the principle remains the same: returning to running requires patience, flexibility, and proper support. With these lessons in mind, let's explore how you can assess if you're ready to increase your activity levels.

Evaluating Your Readiness for Impact Activities

After completing your Twelve-Week *Strong as a Mother* Activity Progression and your Core and Strength Training Program, it's important to evaluate your readiness for more demanding movements. Think of this as your preseason evaluation—a chance to thoroughly assess your foundation before building on it.

THE STRONG AS A MOTHER ASSESSMENT PROTOCOL

General Readiness Indicators

Before increasing your exercise intensity, verify that you:

- Have clearance from your healthcare provider
- Are pain-free during daily activities
- Can comfortably walk for four miles
- Have good balance and stability
- Do not have RED-S

Orthopedic Strength Markers

Whether you are postpartum or not, these benchmarks support running biomechanics and most high-level activities. Being able to successfully complete most of these strength markers should give you the confidence to return to the activities you love with a reduced risk of injury. You should be able to perform the exercises in the following self-assessment.

Self-Assessment Exercises

EXERCISE	FREQUENCY	PAGE
Single-Leg Squat to Runner's Drive	10 reps	248
Full Plank	30 seconds	221
Runner's Toe Taps	10 reps	235
Split-Stance Romanian Deadlifts	10 reps	251
Single-Leg Balance Clock Reaches	85 percent of leg length*	245
Single-Leg Calf Raises (Weighted)	10 reps	247
Runner's Bent-Knee Calf Raises (Weighted)	20 reps	233
Single-Leg Bridges (Weighted)	10 reps per side	246
Side Plank Leg Lifts	10 reps	243
Side Plank Hip Drops	10 reps	227
Modified Copenhagen on Jump Box	30 seconds per side	231
Single-Leg Hops (Forward/Backward)	8 reps	247
Single-Leg Hops (Side-to-Side)	8 reps	247
Scissor Jumps	8 reps	235
Box Jumps	8 reps	211

Note: To measure leg length, sit against a wall, mark your heel location, and measure the distance from wall to heel for Single-Leg Balance Clock Reaches.

Remember, this checklist isn't about perfection—even professional athletes have areas for improvement. Use these benchmarks to identify any areas of your physical fitness that could use additional support as you return to high-level activities. If you find it difficult to complete most of these exercises, carefully consider the benefits and risks of returning to high-level activity, and focus on strengthening your hips and core. It may also be helpful to consult a pelvic floor specialist, especially if you experience leakage, pain, or a sensation of heaviness in your pelvis when running.

Sport-Specific Considerations

Running serves as the foundation for most athletic activities, and the benchmarks included in here support a wide range of sports. However, you may still need additional sport-specific strength assessments. Consider working with healthcare providers who are trained in your particular sport to develop a tailored evaluation and training program.

Guidelines for a Safe Return

Regardless of whether you're returning to running or other high-impact activities, it's important to remember that overuse injuries to the muscles, bones, and ligaments are among the most common setbacks for exercisers. Follow the principles below to help minimize your risk of injuries.

- Listen to your body—modify your exercise routine as needed.
- Exercise every other day at first.
- Focus on form—pregnancy changes have affected your movement patterns.
- Delay speed work until you have sufficient strength and endurance before you add intensity.
- Introduce hill work before speed work.
- Prioritize strength training.
- Change only one variable at a time, such as surface, incline, intensity, speed, volume, or footwear.
- Start with two shorter sessions and one longer session per week.
- Stop if you experience pain greater than a 3 on a scale of 1–10 during activity.
- Reduce your exercise volume or intensity if pain persists 24 hours after exercising.
- Progress gradually when comfortable.

A Note on the Baby Boost

Some athletes report an improvement in VO2 max (the maximum amount of oxygen the body can utilize during intense exercise) postpartum, a phenomenon often referred to as the "baby boost." However, since VO2 max isn't the only—or necessarily the best—predictor of performance, approach this cautiously, and:

- Factor in the energy demands of nursing

- Account for sleep patterns and stress levels
- Ensure your nutritional intake supports the demands of sports and motherhood.
- Remember, you should gradually build up your activity level to avoid physical and emotional setbacks.

Choosing Your Activities

Different activities require different approaches. Running, for instance, demands careful attention to progression due to its impact forces. Here are some tips for your return to running or other high-intensity activities.

FOR RUNNERS

- Start with run/walk intervals.
- Prioritize form over speed.
- Use recovery days purposefully.
- Consider working with a running coach.
- Incorporate cross-training.

FOR ALL ACTIVITIES

- Build bone health with varied movements.
- Include at least one cross-training session each week.
- Monitor pelvic floor symptoms.
- Track your energy levels.
- Continue strength training.

FROM THE PRO
Jessica's Training Insight

Success isn't just about meeting physical benchmarks—it's about establishing sustainable patterns that honor both your athletic goals and your new role as a mother. Sometimes this means redefining what progress looks like.

Remember that every postpartum journey is unique. While these guidelines provide a framework, your personal path may require adjustments. Working with healthcare providers who understand both postpartum recovery and athletic performance can help you navigate this transition successfully.

CHAPTER 21

Your Lifelong Wellness Journey

The work you've put in during pregnancy and your postpartum period has laid a strong foundation for lifelong health. As you move beyond the fourth trimester, it's important to shift your focus to creating sustainable patterns that support your heart, bones, and overall well-being for decades to come.

STRONG BONES FOR LIFE

The postpartum period is a critical time for your bone health. Similar to menopause, the drop in estrogen during this phase affects your muscles, ligaments, and bones. Understanding this shift can help you protect your bone density over the long term.

The Bone-Building Challenge

While many people believe that running and strength training are the best activities for building bone density, activities that move your body in multiple directions actually provide greater benefits.

Consider adding one or two of these bone-building activities to your routine:

- Basketball
- Impact aerobics
- Dancing
- Gymnastics
- Tennis
- Jumping rope

Important Note: Pregnancy and nursing can affect bone density. If returning to high-volume running, consider getting regular bone density scans from your healthcare provider. The key is to progress gradually, especially when your estrogen levels are low and your bones need extra protection.

HEART HEALTH FOR LIFE

Many of us know that cardiovascular exercise supports heart health, but understanding why it matters, particularly during the postpartum years, can help motivate you to move consistently.

Regular cardio helps regulate hormones, supports good mental health, and lays the foundation for lifelong wellness—benefits that will support you as you navigate the physical and emotional demands of motherhood.

Making Movement Matter

The American Heart Association recommends 150 minutes of moderate activity or 75 minutes of vigorous activity weekly, ideally a combination of both types. These aren't just arbitrary numbers—this amount of movement helps:

• Regulate blood pressure
• Strengthen your heart muscle
• Support healthy cholesterol levels
• Improve sleep quality
• Boost energy levels
• Enhance mood
• Reduce anxiety
• Maintain a healthy weight
• Support bone density

These goals are more achievable than you might think. Exercise doesn't require a gym membership or dedicated workout time. Movement can be woven into your daily life in ways that enhance quality time with your family rather than competing with it.

Finding Your Level

Moderate activities get your heart pumping while still allowing you to hold a conversation. Examples include:

• Hiking local trails
• Playing doubles tennis
• Mowing the lawn
• Participating in water aerobics
• Taking a brisk walk

Vigorous activities make conversation challenging. Examples include:

• Running or jogging
• Jump rope sessions
• Cycling on hilly terrain
• Singles tennis matches

BUILDING STRENGTH FOR YOUR FUTURE

The years between pregnancy and menopause, which are roughly between the ages of thirty-five and fifty, offer a window for building muscle mass and bone density. This investment in strength training helps:

• Maintain a healthy body weight
• Regulate blood pressure
• Stabilize your blood sugar
• Build muscle reserves for your post-menopausal years

The good news? You don't need complicated routines or expensive equipment.

Focus on:

- Training all major muscle groups twice a week
- Working your legs, hips, back, abdomen, chest, shoulders, and arms
- Completing one set of 8 to 12 reps per area
- Choosing weights or resistances that make the last few repetitions challenging
- Using whatever tools you have—weights, resistance bands, or even household items

LISTENING TO YOUR BODY'S SIGNALS

While building strength is important, it's equally vital to pay attention to how your body responds. If you experience symptoms such as urinary urgency, leakage, or pelvic heaviness, consider:

- Moving intense workouts to a different time of day
- Allowing adequate pelvic rest after challenging sessions
- Working with your healthcare provider to modify activities or provide interventions as needed

Pay particular attention if you find yourself:

- Skipping workouts due to symptoms
- Reducing intensity more than you'd like
- Shortening your workout duration
- Exercising less frequently than desired

Symptom-related changes in your exercise habits warrant a conversation with your healthcare provider, as they often have solutions that can help you stay active while supporting your pelvic health.

Remember, the habits you establish now will help support lifelong wellness. By combining bone-building activities, cardiovascular exercise, and strength training, you're investing in your health—not just for the next few years, but for decades to come.

Strong as a Mother

Throughout this book we've explored pregnancy and postpartum recovery through the lens of training as an athlete—not because every mother is an Olympian, but because every mother deserves the same thoughtful attention to preparation, performance, and recovery. As we conclude our time together, let's take a moment to reflect on the fundamental principles that guide you on your journey through motherhood.

SET A STRONG FOUNDATION

Think back to the early chapters where we discussed the importance of preparation. Just as an athlete wouldn't show up unprepared on race day, the groundwork you lay during pregnancy significantly impacts your postpartum recovery. Every small choice—whether it's a pelvic floor exercise, a mindful movement, or a moment spent learning about your changing body—adds to your strength. These seemingly minor actions accumulate, creating a robust framework that will support you through pregnancy, birth, and beyond.

FROM THE PRO
Shannon's Perspective on Preparation

As an athlete, I learned that success comes from consistent, thoughtful preparation. Motherhood is no different. The time you invest in understanding and supporting your body during pregnancy not only benefits you in the immediate postpartum period but also pays dividends throughout your entire motherhood journey.

FROM THE PRO
Jessica's Perspective on Preparation

Postpartum fitness isn't about what we do after baby arrives. It's what we do during pregnancy that sets us up for success. We are twice as likely to return to the activities we love if we stay active during pregnancy. Every moment you choose movement becomes a building blocks in your foundation of strength. In that consistency is life-long health.

BE PROACTIVE

Throughout this book, we've emphasized the intricate relationship between your core, hips, and pelvic floor. These aren't separate muscle groups; they're a team—working together to support every movement you make. To support these muscles, finding balance is key. This means strengthening your stabilizing muscles while maintaining the flexibility needed for birth, developing quick-response and endurance capabilities in your pelvic floor, and coordinating all these elements to move efficiently and confidently.

This balanced approach becomes even more important when we consider some sobering statistics. Research shows that without proper intervention, 92 percent of women who experience leakage at twelve weeks postpartum will still face this challenge five years later. A weakened pelvic floor isn't just a hormone issue that resolves once you stop nursing—it's a call to action for proactive pelvic health care.

THE FOUR PILLARS OF LIFELONG STRENGTH

As you continue your motherhood journey, remember the four essential factors that support effective exercise and overall wellness:

- **Intensity:** Understanding how hard to work

- **Frequency:** Knowing how often to train
- **Duration:** Determining how long to sustain an activity
- **Work/Rest Ratio:** Balancing effort with recovery

These principles provide a framework for maintaining strength and wellness throughout motherhood. They will guide you not just through pregnancy and postpartum recovery, but throughout your entire life—including perimenopause, menopause, and beyond.

HONOR YOUR JOURNEY

Society often imposes rigid timelines and expectations for pregnancy, birth, and postpartum recovery. You might feel pressured to bounce back, return to previous activities by certain dates, or meet others' definitions of success. But remember this fundamental truth: your journey is uniquely yours. The timeline that works for one mother might not work for another, and that's not just okay—it's exactly as it should be.

FROM THE PRO
Jessica's Insight on Individual Progress

In my practice, I've seen how comparing recovery timelines can create unnecessary stress. The key isn't reaching certain milestones by specific dates—it's making consistent progress while honoring your body's signals and needs, as well as your baby's.

MOVE FORWARD WITH CONFIDENCE

As you continue your motherhood journey, remember the essential principles below.

Trust Your Foundation

The knowledge and strength you've built during pregnancy will serve as your foundation for years to come. Understanding your body's needs and capabilities helps you make informed decisions about movement and recovery.

Stay Active Your Way

Choose activities that bring you joy and energy. Whether it's running, swimming, strength training, or gentle movement, the best exercise is the one you'll stick with. Modify your activities as needed but keep moving in ways that feel right for your body.

Maintain Balance

Just as your pelvic floor needs both length and strength for optimal function, your overall approach to movement and motherhood thrives on balance—balance between effort and rest, strength and flexibility, and between meeting your needs and caring for your family.

Seek Support When Needed

Seeking help isn't a sign of weakness—it's a strategy for success. Whether it's working with a pelvic floor specialist, joining a postpartum exercise group, or connecting with other mothers, support enriches your journey.

YOUR CONTINUING STRENGTH

You're embarking on your own journey to being Strong as a Mother. Whether you're an experienced athlete or new to movement, your journey matters. The strength you build now—physical, mental, and emotional—creates a foundation for your own well-being and that of generations to come.

You have the knowledge, tools, and most importantly, strength within you to thrive through every stage of motherhood. Remember, becoming strong as a mother isn't about reaching a finish line—it's about embracing the ongoing journey of growth through every stage of life.

Join the @4TwoMom Community

You've completed the programs, learned the techniques, and built your foundation of strength. Now it's time to connect with others who share your commitment to being strong as a mother.

Remember, you're not alone on this journey! We invite you to join our @4TwoMom community, where you can:

- Share your goals and celebrate your victories
- Find support and encouragement from other moms
- Multiply your joys and divide your concerns

Whether you're navigating your first pregnancy or adding to your family, motherhood is an incredible adventure that's even better when shared. Let's embark on this journey together and cheer each other on every step of the way!

Exercise Reference Guide

This comprehensive reference section serves as your trusted exercise guide throughout your pregnancy and postpartum journey. While the structured programs elsewhere in this book note which exercises to learn each week, this section provides the detailed instructions, form cues, and modifications for every movement you'll encounter.

We've organized this reference guide with intention. You'll find the exercise fundamentals, starting positions, and essential reminders at the beginning because these elements form the foundation of safe, effective movement during this transformative time in your body.

The pelvic floor exercises follow these fundamentals because they represent the literal foundation of your core system. As you've learned, optimal movement begins with pelvic stability and proper breathing mechanics. These specialized exercises may appear simple, but they form the basis of both your recovery and long-term strength. It's important to master them before beginning the other trimester programs.

Next, you'll find the alphabetized exercise library. This organization allows you to quickly locate specific movements while ensuring you approach them with the proper foundational knowledge. For higher-level exercises like plyometrics, consult your healthcare team. In the third trimester, place a pillow behind your upper back to improve blood flow to your baby when performing exercises or activities on your back. Also, if balance is a challenge, find something to hold onto for stability.

Whether you're referencing these pages during your first trimester or deep into your postpartum recovery, take time to revisit the fundamentals regularly. As your body changes, your relationship with these movements will evolve, and returning to these principles will support your journey toward strength in motherhood.

EXERCISE FUNDAMENTALS

Understanding these core principles ensures that every movement you perform supports your changing body while building sustainable strength. These fundamentals apply universally across all exercises in this guide.

Breathing

START: Lie on your back with knees bent, and your feet flat on the floor.

MOVEMENT:

1 Place one hand on your chest and the other on your belly.

2 Inhale slowly, allowing your belly to rise while expanding your rib cage.

3 Exhale naturally, feeling your belly fall without forcing or straining.

4 Continue for 2–3 minutes, focusing on the rhythm and quality of each breath.

EQUIPMENT
• Mat

FOCUS
• Notice the length of each breath
• Feel expansion in all directions
• Keep shoulders relaxed

Core Activation Technique

START: Begin in any comfortable position (lying, seated, or standing).

MOVEMENT:

1 Inhale deeply through your nose, allowing your belly to expand.

2 Exhale and draw your sternum (breastbone) down toward your belly button about 1 inch.

3 Simultaneously lift your pubic bone toward your belly button.

4 Pull your belly button toward your spine with 30-50 percent effort.

5 Maintain normal breathing while holding this engagement.

EQUIPMENT
• Mat or chair

FOCUS
• Keep pelvic floor gently activated
• Breathe normally
• Avoid holding your breath

STARTING POSITIONS

How you begin a movement largely determines its safety and effectiveness. These poses establish proper alignment and create the starting postions for the exercises in this book. When in doubt, always return to these fundamental starting positions before beginning any movement.

Lying

EQUIPMENT
• Mat
• Pillow (optional)

FOCUS
• Keep spine in neutral position
• Relax shoulders
• Use pillow behind upper back after first trimester

START: Find a comfortable surface with enough space to lie down fully.

MOVEMENT:

1 Lie on your back with your knees bent.

2 Place your feet flat on the floor, hip-width apart.

3 Engage your core using the Core Activation technique.

4 Rest arms comfortably at your sides or on your abdomen.

Side Lying

EQUIPMENT
• Mat
• Pillow (optional)

FOCUS
• Keep spine neutral
• Stack shoulders directly above each other
• Avoid twisting

START: Find a comfortable surface with enough space to lie down fully.

MOVEMENT:

1 Lie on your side with knees bent at a 90-degree angle.

2 Stack your hips directly on top of each other.

3 Use pillows between knees and under head for comfort if needed.

4 Engage your core using the Core Activation technique.

Kneeling Side Plank

START: Begin in side-lying position with knees bent at 90-degree angle.

MOVEMENT:

1 Stack your hips on top of each other.

2 Position your forearm slightly under your shoulder.

3 Engage your core and lift your hips up off the floor.

4 Create a straight line from your knees to your shoulders.

EQUIPMENT
• Mat

FOCUS
• Keep hips level
• Avoid arching back
• Press forearm firmly into the mat

Side Plank

START: Begin in side-lying position with legs extended.

MOVEMENT:

1 Stack your hips on top of each other.

2 Position your forearm slightly under your shoulder.

3 Engage your core and lift your hips up toward the ceiling.

4 Create a straight line from your ankles to your shoulders.

EQUIPMENT
• Mat

FOCUS
• Keep hips level
• Avoid arching back
• Maintain strong shoulder position

Four Point

START: Find a comfortable surface with enough cushioning for your hands and knees.

MOVEMENT:

1 Start on hands and knees, with knees bent at 90-degree angle.

2 Position hands directly under shoulders, your fingers pointing your forward.

3 Press into your shoulder blades without arching your back.

4 Keep elbows slightly bent and pull hands back toward feet without moving them.

5 Engage your core.

EQUIPMENT
• Mat

FOCUS
• The harder you pull back your hands, the more you engage your abdominals
• Keep your back flat

Bear Plank

EQUIPMENT
• Mat

FOCUS
• Keep hips level
• Avoid sagging in lower back
• Pull hands toward feet without moving them

START: Begin in the four-point position.

MOVEMENT:

1 Position hands directly under shoulders, your fingers pointing forward.

2 Lift both knees off the ground by one inch.

3 Keep your back flat and knees bent.

4 Engage your core throughout the hold.

Seated

EQUIPMENT
• Chair
• Stability ball (optional)

FOCUS
• Maintain neutral spine
• Avoid slouching
• Keep weight evenly distributed on sitting bones

START: Find a sturdy chair or stability ball.

MOVEMENT:

1 Sit at the front edge of the chair or ball.

2 Keep your feet flat on the floor, hip-width apart.

3 Stack shoulders over hips and lengthen through the spine.

4 Engage your core.

Standing

EQUIPMENT
None

FOCUS
• Keep chest lifted
• Relax shoulders
• Maintain a gentle knee bend for stability

START: Find a clear space where you can stand comfortably.

MOVEMENT:

1 Stand with feet slightly wider than shoulder-width apart.

2 Point feet in a comfortable position.

3 Divide weight evenly between the front of heels and balls of feet.

4 Bend your knees slightly and lift arches.

5 Engage your core.

EXERCISE REMINDERS

These essential reminders serve as your movement mantras throughout pregnancy and postpartum recovery. Post them where you'll see them during workouts, or mentally review them before beginning your practice. They'll guide you toward mindful, effective movement that honors your body's changing needs.

When performing any exercise in this program, keep these key principles in mind:

1 RIB CAGE POSITION: Keep muscles around lower ribs engaged to prevent flaring.

2 PELVIC POSITION: Maintain a neutral pelvis position (not tilted excessively forward or back).

3 BREATHING: Breathe naturally throughout all movements, never holding your breath.

4 CORE ENGAGEMENT: Maintain gentle core activation using the technique on page 199.

5 FORM PRIORITY: Always prioritize proper form over completing more repetitions.

6 MODIFICATION: Adjust exercises as needed to accommodate your changing body.

7 PROGRESSION: Advance only when you can maintain proper form throughout the exercise, adding weights and resistance bands as appropriate.

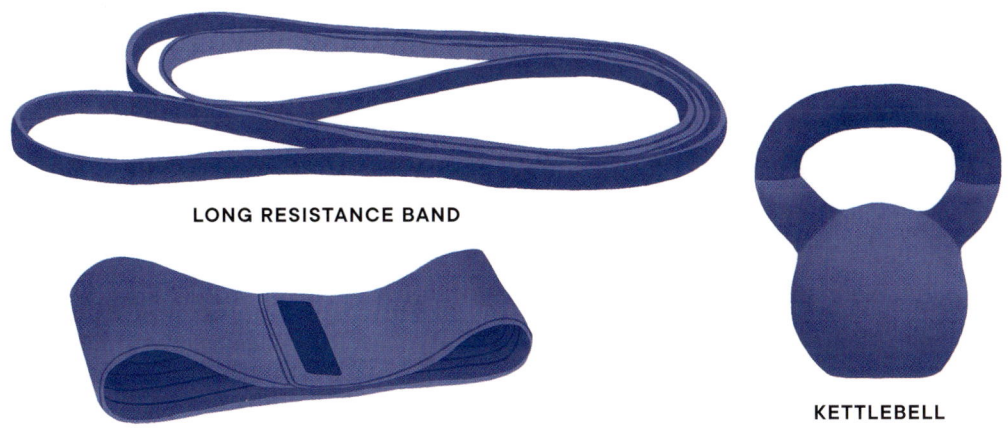

LONG RESISTANCE BAND

LOOP BAND

KETTLEBELL

PELVIC FLOOR EXERCISES

As you've learned, the pelvic floor represents the foundation of your core system, supporting your organs, stabilizing your pelvis, and playing a crucial role in continence and sexual function. These specialized exercises build awareness and function in this vital muscle group. While they may seem subtle, their impact on your overall recovery and strength is profound. Master these movements first, as they inform all other exercises in this guide.

Static Hold

EQUIPMENT
• Chair or mat

FOCUS
• Maintain normal breathing
• Keep shoulders relaxed
• Avoid tensing buttocks or inner thighs

START: Sit comfortably with good posture or lie on your back with knees bent.

MOVEMENT:

1 Round your back slightly, then gently tighten the muscles that close your anus, as if trying to hold in gas.

2 Arch back slightly and contract muscles around the clitoris and urethra.

3 Hold at 30-50 percent strength for target duration (work up to 33 seconds).

4 Release completely and rest briefly between repetitions, alternating between Steps 1 and 2.

Quick Flicks

EQUIPMENT
• Chair or mat

FOCUS
• Maintain rhythmic pattern
• Keep buttocks relaxed
• Breathe normally

START: Sit comfortably with good posture or lie on your back with knees bent.

MOVEMENT:

1 Arch your back slightly.

2 Tighten pelvic floor muscles for 1 second, focusing on urethra area.

3 Relax completely for 1 second before repeating.

Elevators

START: Sit comfortably with good posture or lie on your back with knees bent.

MOVEMENT:

1 Start fully relaxed (ground floor).

2 Contract to 25 percent strength (first floor), pause briefly.

3 Increase to 50 percent (second floor), then 75 percent (third floor), then 100 percent (top floor).

4 Descend in reverse order: 75 percent, 50 percent, 25 percent, fully relaxed.

EQUIPMENT
• **Chair or mat**

FOCUS
• **Move smoothly between levels**
• **Breathe normally**
• **Maintain good posture**

Half-Holds with 3 Quick Flicks

START: Sit comfortably with good posture or lie on your back with knees bent.

MOVEMENT:

1 Contract pelvic floor to 50 percent strength and hold.

2 While maintaining the 50 percent contraction, perform 3 quick flicks to 100 percent strength.

3 Return to 50 percent after each flick.

4 Fully release and relax after the third flick.

EQUIPMENT
• **Chair or mat**

FOCUS
• **Maintain baseline 50 percent hold throughout**
• **Breathe normally**
• **Keep abdomen relaxed**

Bearing Down

START: Sit comfortably with good posture or lie on your back with knees bent.

MOVEMENT:

1 Breathe deeply into your belly, allowing it to expand.

2 As you feel air move downward, consciously relax your anus.

3 Follow your breath—relax on inhale, return to baseline on exhale.

→ **SEE ALSO:** Chapter 14: Essential Birthing Techniques, page 107.

Note: Bearing Down is beneficial for delivery preparation and activities like inserting a tampon, relaxing for intercourse, and easing bowel movements.

EQUIPMENT
• **Chair or mat**

FOCUS
• **Focus on relaxation more than pushing**
• **Keep neck and jaw relaxed**
• **Allow natural expansion**

ALPHABETICAL EXERCISE GUIDE

Now that you've established the foundational principles, positions, and pelvic floor awareness, you're ready to explore the complete exercise library. Each movement includes detailed instructions, form cues, and trimester-specific modifications to support your changing body.

70/30 Bridges

EQUIPMENT
• Mat

FOCUS
• Maintain weight distribution
• Keep core engaged
• Control the movement

START: Lying position

MOVEMENT:

1 Shift 70 percent of your weight toward one foot.

2 Raise your hips until your knees, hips, and shoulders form a straight line, keeping your rib muscles engaged. Avoid arching your back.

3 Lower hips back to ground with control.

4 Complete 10 repetitions per side, 1-2 sets.

70/30 Calf Raises

EQUIPMENT
• Stable surface

FOCUS
• Maintain weight distribution
• Control the movement
• Keep arches lifted

START: Standing position near a stable surface

MOVEMENT:

1 Shift 70 percent of weight onto one leg.

2 Rise onto balls of feet while maintaining the 70/30 weight distribution.

3 Hold for one second at top position.

4 Lower with control back to starting position.

5 Complete 10 repetitions per side, 1-2 sets.

70/30 Squats

START: Standing position

MOVEMENT:

1 Shift 70 percent of your weight onto your working leg.

2 Lower into mini squat position while maintaining the weight distribution.

3 Return to standing position with control.

4 Complete 10 repetitions per side, 1-2 sets.

EQUIPMENT
None

FOCUS
- Maintain weight distribution
- Keep working knee aligned
- Avoid arching back

Arch Lifts

START: Standing position

MOVEMENT:

1 Press big toes into the ground.

2 Lift arches and hold for 1 second.

3 Slowly lower arches back down, controlling the movement.

4 Complete 20 repetitions, 1-2 sets.

EQUIPMENT
None

FOCUS
- Keep toes grounded
- Control the movement
- Maintain balance

Arm Lifts

START: Lying position

MOVEMENT:

1 Engage your core to stabilize your torso.

2 Lift one arm up and over while keeping back flat and rib muscles engaged.

3 Move arm only as far as your core can maintain engagement and back stays flat.

4 Return to starting position with control before alternating arms.

5 Complete 10 repetitions per side, 2 sets.

EQUIPMENT
- Mat

FOCUS
- Keep back flat throughout
- Engage rib muscles
- Control the movement

Arm Lifts (Weighted)

EQUIPMENT
• 4-6 pound weights
• Mat

FOCUS
• Control the weight throughout
• Maintain stable torso
• Keep shoulder blades on the mat

START: Lying position

MOVEMENT:

1 In one arm, hold a weight at chest level.

2 Lift arm while keeping back flat and ribs engaged.

3 Move arm only as far as your core remains engaged and back stays flat.

4 Return to starting position with control before alternating arms.

5 Complete 10 repetitions per side, 2 sets.

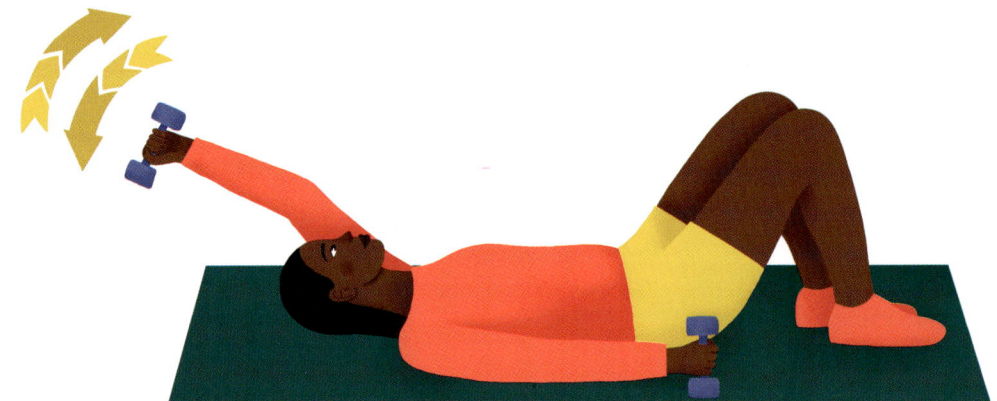

Bear Plank Knee Taps

EQUIPMENT
• Mat

FOCUS
• Keep back flat throughout
• Maintain stable hips
• Control the movement
• Engage core throughout

START: Four-point position

MOVEMENT:

1 Press chest toward ceiling to engage shoulder blades.

2 Lift knees slightly off ground while keeping back flat.

3 Lower one knee to tap the ground, then lift it back up.

4 Alternate sides, completing 10 repetitions per side, 1-2 sets.

Bear Plank Leg Lifts

START: Four-point position

MOVEMENT:

1 Press chest toward ceiling to engage shoulder blades.

2 Lift knees slightly off ground while keeping back flat.

3 Lift one leg behind you, straightening the knee.

4 Alternate sides, completing 10 repetitions per side, 1-2 sets.

EQUIPMENT
• Mat

FOCUS
• Keep back flat
• Lift leg only to height that maintains neutral spine
• Control the movement
• Engage core throughout

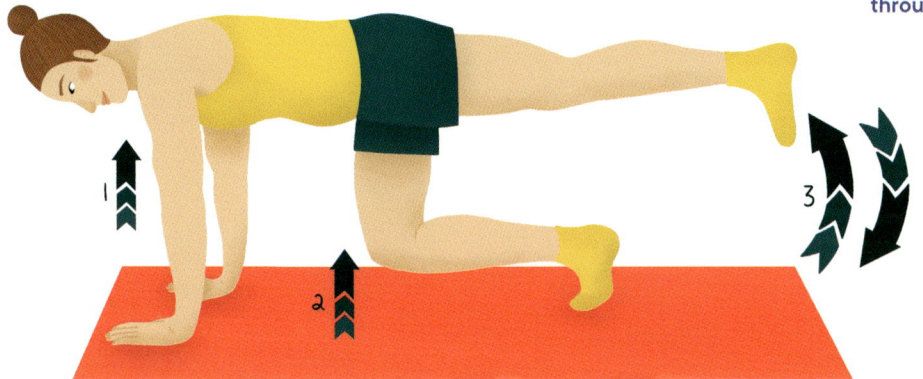

Bent-Knee 70/30 Calf Raises

START: Standing position with both knees bent at a 30-degree angle

MOVEMENT:

1 Shift 70 percent of weight onto one leg.

2 Rise onto balls of feet, keeping knees bent at 30-degree angle.

3 Hold the top position for one second.

4 Lower slowly over 3-second count back to starting position.

5 Complete 20 repetitions per side, 1-2 sets.

EQUIPMENT
• Stable surface for support

FOCUS
• Maintain weight distribution
• Keep knees bent
• Control the movement

Bent-Knee Calf Raises

EQUIPMENT
• Stable surface for support

FOCUS
• Maintain bent knees throughout
• Control the lowering phase
• Keep arches lifted

START: Standing position with both knees bent at a 30-degree angle

MOVEMENT:

1 Rise onto balls of feet, keeping knees bent at 30-degree angle.

2 Hold top position for one second.

3 Lower slowly over 3-second count back to starting position.

4 Complete 20 repetitions, 1-2 sets.

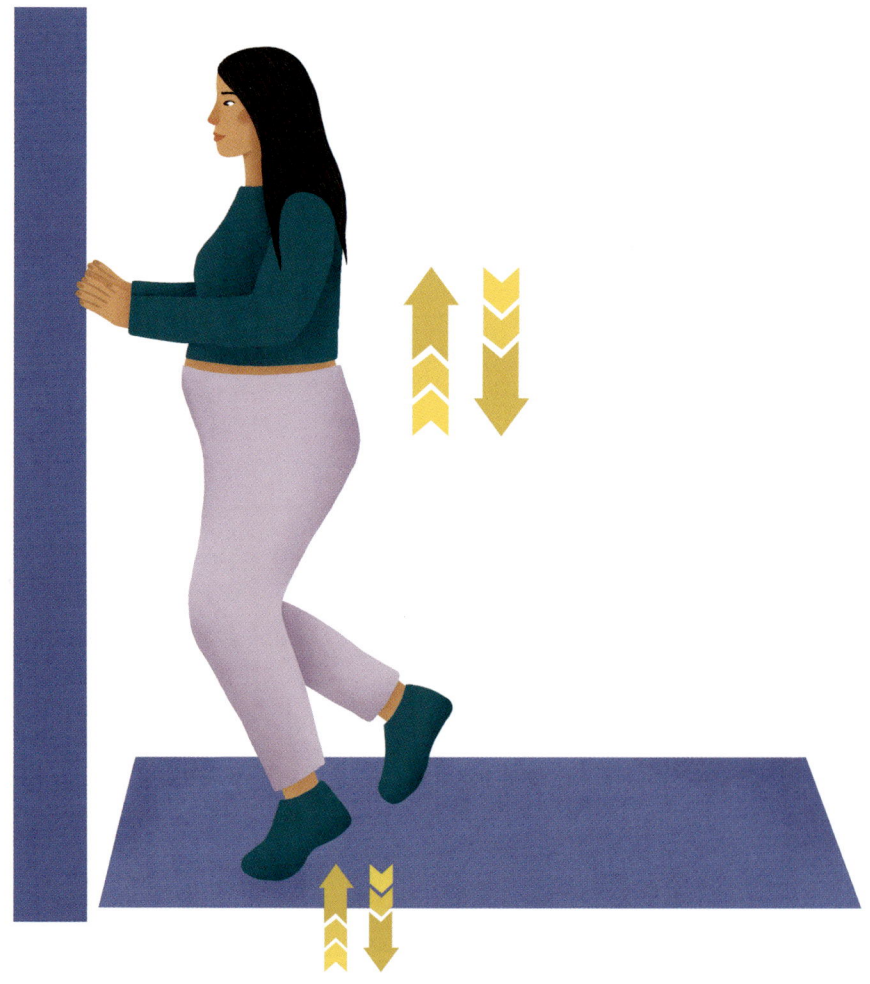

BENT-KNEE SINGLE-LEG CALF RAISES

Bent-Knee Calf Stretch

START: Standing position facing wall with hands at shoulder height for support

MOVEMENT:

1 Step back with one leg, keeping both knees slightly bent.

2 Lean forward until you feel deep stretch in back calf.

3 Hold for 30 seconds, maintaining back heel contact with floor.

4 Complete 1-2 sets per side.

EQUIPMENT
• **Wall**

FOCUS
• **Maintain bent knees throughout**
• **Keep arches lifted**

Bent-Knee Single-Leg Calf Raises

START: Standing position with both knees bent at a 30-degree angle

MOVEMENT:

1 Shift all your weight onto one leg, keeping the non- working leg off the ground.

2 Rise onto ball of working foot, keeping knee bent at 30-degree angle.

3 Hold top position for one second.

4 Lower slowly over 3-second count back to starting position.

5 Complete 20 repetitions per side, 1-2 sets.

EQUIPMENT
• **Stable surface, weights (optional)**

FOCUS
• **Maintain bent knee position**
• **Control the movement**
• **Keep arch lifted**

Box Jumps

START: Standing position in front of a low jump box or step

MOVEMENT:

1 Lower into slight squat position.

2 Jump onto the box, keeping knees aligned and landing softly.

3 Step back down with control.

4 Complete 8 repetitions, 2 sets.

EQUIPMENT
• **Low jump box or step**

FOCUS
• **Land softly with bent knees**
• **Align knees over toes**

Box Taps

EQUIPMENT
• Low jump box or step

FOCUS
• Maintain upright posture
• Stay light on feet

START: Standing position in front of a low jump box or step

MOVEMENT:

1   Quickly tap one foot on the edge of the box.

2   Alternate feet while maintaining upright posture.

3   Keep a steady rhythm and maintain balance.

4   Complete 8 repetitions per side, 2 sets.

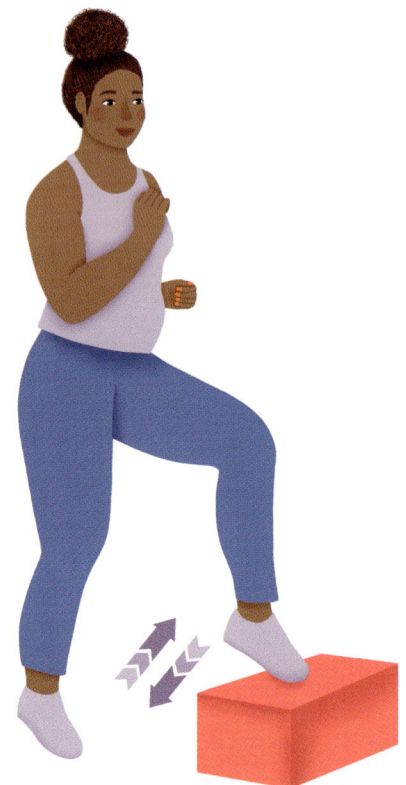

Bridges

EQUIPMENT
• Mat

FOCUS
• Distribute pressure evenly across both feet
• Avoid arching lower back
• Engage glutes and rib muscles

START: Lying position

MOVEMENT:

1   Engage your core and press through feet to lift hips.

2   Raise hips until knees, hips, and shoulders form a straight line.

3   Keep rib muscles engaged and avoid arching back.

4   Lower hips back to ground with control.

5   Complete 10 repetitions, 1-2 sets.

Bridges with Heel Lifts

START: Lying position

MOVEMENT:

1. Lift your hips into bridge position.

2. Lift one heel off the ground while keeping knee bent.

3. Keep hips level as you lower heel back to ground with control.

4. Alternate heels, then return to starting position.

5. Complete 10 repetitions per side, 1-2 sets.

EQUIPMENT
- Mat

FOCUS
- Maintain level hips throughout
- Keep core engaged
- Control the movement

Calf Raises

START: Standing position near a stable surface

MOVEMENT:

1. Rise onto balls of feet while lifting arches.

2. Hold for one second at top position.

3. Lower with control, taking 1 second to return to starting position.

4. Complete 10 repetitions, 1-2 sets.

EQUIPMENT
- Stable surface for support

FOCUS
- Lift arches while raising
- Control the descent
- Maintain balance

Calf Stretch

START: Standing position facing a wall with hands pushing against it at shoulder height

MOVEMENT:

1. Step back with one leg, keeping it straight with heel on floor.

2. Bend front knee until you feel stretch in back calf.

3. Hold for 30 seconds, maintaining back heel contact with floor.

4. Complete 1-2 sets per side.

EQUIPMENT
- Wall

FOCUS
- Keep back leg straight
- Maintain heel contact with floor
- Feel gentle stretch

Child's Pose Stretch

EQUIPMENT
• Mat
• Pillows (optional)

FOCUS
• Allow pelvic floor
  to relax
• Breathe deeply
• Use pillows for
  support if needed

START: Four-point position with knees wider than shoulders

MOVEMENT:

1 Round upper back, expanding ribs as you inhale.

2 Allow pelvic floor to lengthen.

3 Push hips back toward heels.

4 Repeat with hands shifted right then left for variation.

5 Hold 30 seconds in each position, 1-2 sets.

Core Curl Ups

EQUIPMENT
• Mat

FOCUS
• Keep back flat
• Maintain core
  engagement
• Control the
  movement

START: Lying position

MOVEMENT:

1 Position hands behind head.

2 Tuck chin toward chest.

3 Lift shoulder blades 4-5 inches from ground while keeping back flat.

4 Hold for 5 seconds.

5 Lower shoulders with control, maintaining proper form.

6 Complete 10 repetitions, 1-2 sets.

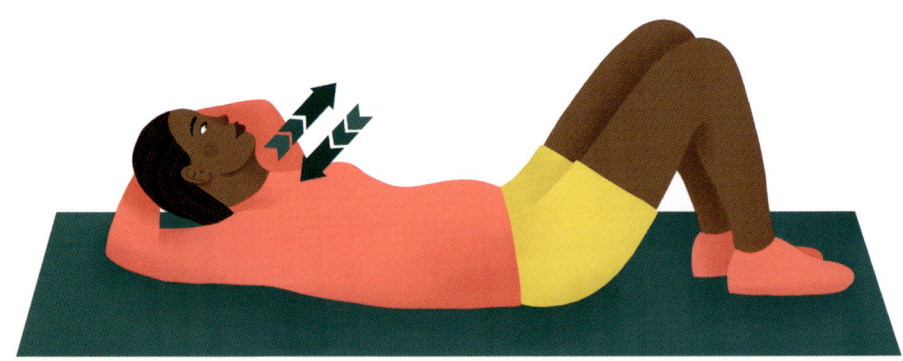

Core Curl Ups (Banded)

START: Lying position with resistance band anchored behind you

MOVEMENT:

1 Hold band near your ears while supporting your neck, creating tension by pulling toward you.

2 Tuck chin toward chest.

3 Lift shoulder blades 4-5 inches from ground while maintaining band tension.

4 Hold for 5 seconds.

5 Lower shoulders with control, maintaining proper form.

6 Complete 10 repetitions, 1-2 sets.

EQUIPMENT
• Long resistance band
• Secure anchor point
• Mat

FOCUS
• Maintain band tension throughout
• Keep back flat
• Control the movement
• Engage core throughout

Core Engagement Holds

START: Lying position

MOVEMENT:

1 Engage your core by gently drawing your navel toward your spine.

2 Hold this engagement for 5 seconds while breathing normally.

3 Release completely between repetitions.

4 Repeat for 10 repetitions, 2 sets.

EQUIPMENT
• Mat

FOCUS
• Maintain normal breathing
• Avoid tilting pelvis
• Feel muscles gently working

Counter Stretch

START: Standing position with hands placed on a countertop

MOVEMENT:

1 Round upper back, expanding ribs as you inhale.

2 Allow pelvic floor to lengthen.

3 Push hips backward, creating length in spine.

4 With each exhale, inch fingers forward to deepen stretch.

5 Repeat with hands shifted right then left.

6 Hold 30 seconds in each position, 1-2 sets.

EQUIPMENT
• Countertop or stable surface

FOCUS
• Keep knees soft
• Allow pelvic floor to relax
• Focus on upper back stretch

Diagonal Pulls (Banded)

START: Standing position with band secured under one foot, holding opposite end in opposite hand

MOVEMENT:

1 Position band across body with palm facing toward belly.

2 Draw shoulder blade down and in.

3 Lift arm up and out, ending with palm facing forward.

4 Return to starting position with control.

5 Complete 10 repetitions per side, 1-2 sets.

Double-Leg Hops (Forward/Backward)

START: Standing position in back corner of target square

MOVEMENT:

1 Jump forward over the line, landing softly on balls of feet.

2 Jump straight back while maintaining control.

3 Keep movements quick and light, staying close to the line.

4 Complete 8 repetitions, 2 sets.

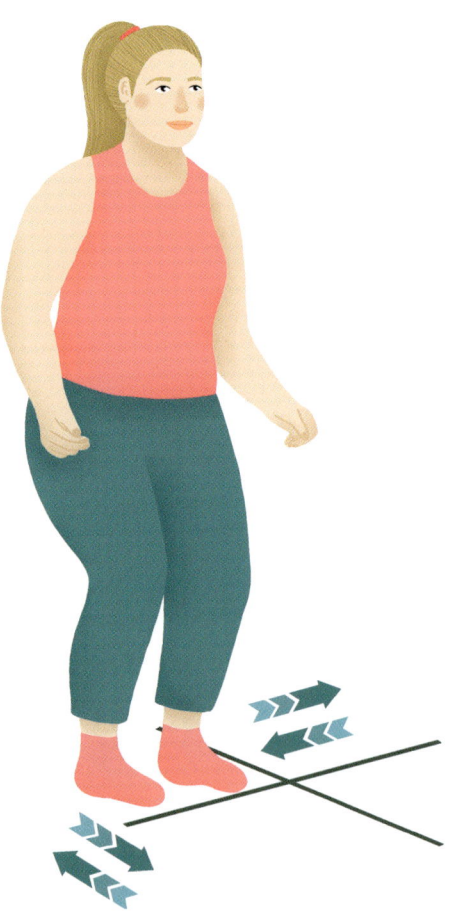

Double-Leg Hops (Side-to-Side)

START: Standing position in back corner of target square

MOVEMENT:

1 Jump sideways over the line, landing softly on balls of feet.

2 Return to starting position immediately while maintaining control.

3 Keep movements quick and light, staying close to the line.

4 Complete 8 repetitions, 2 sets.

EQUIPMENT
- Target square (tape or markers)

FOCUS
- Land softly
- Control movements
- Stay balanced throughout

Dynamic Adductor Stretch

START: Standing position with heel resting on elevated surface, toes pointing up

MOVEMENT:

1 Elevate your leg high enough to feel a stretch in your inner thigh.

2 Gently rock foot side to side 10-15 times.

3 Keep toe pointing up and reach hand along extended leg 10-15 times.

4 Ensure hips face forward throughout movement.

5 Complete 10-15 reps per movement, per side, 1-2 sets

EQUIPMENT
- Stable surface like bench or stool

FOCUS
- Keep hips facing forward
- Maintain balance
- Adjust height based on flexibility

Foam Roller Upper-Back Stretch

EQUIPMENT
• Foam roller
• Mat

FOCUS
• Support head throughout
• Keep core engaged
• Focus on breathing into tight areas

START: Lying position with foam roller placed horizontally under shoulder blades

MOVEMENT:

1 Bend your knees, keeping your feet flat on floor.

2 Supporting your head with your hands, allow upper back to gently extend over roller for three breaths.

3 Move roller down spine one inch at a time.

4 Repeat from shoulder blades to bra line.

5 Complete 1-2 sets.

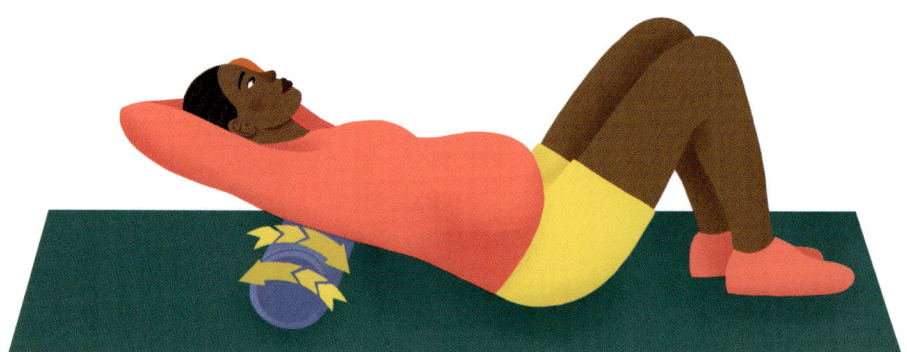

Forward Lunges

EQUIPMENT
• Mat
• Weights (optional)

FOCUS
• Align front knee over ankle
• Keep pelvis level
• Control the movement

START: Standing position

MOVEMENT:

1 Step forward with one foot, keeping feet hip-width apart.

2 Bend both knees until front knee forms a 45-degree angle.

3 Push through front foot to return to starting position.

4 Keep hips and pelvis level throughout the movement.

5 Complete 10 repetitions per side, 1-2 sets.

Four-Point Arm Lifts

START: Four-point position

MOVEMENT:

1 Lift one arm straight forward, aligning with ear.

2 Keep hips stable and shoulders level throughout.

3 Lower arm back to starting position with control.

4 Alternate sides, completing 10 repetitions per side, 2 sets.

EQUIPMENT
• Mat

FOCUS
• Maintain stable pelvis and keep core engaged
• Keep shoulders level
• Control the movement

Four-Point Leg Lifts

START: Four-point position

MOVEMENT:

1 Extend one leg straight back, lifting slightly off ground.

2 Keep hips stable and shoulders level throughout.

3 Lower leg back to starting position with control.

4 Alternate sides, completing 10 repetitions per side, 2 sets.

EQUIPMENT
• Mat

FOCUS
• Maintain stable pelvis and keep core engaged
• Keep hips level
• Lift only to height that preserves alignment

Four-Point Opposite Arm and Leg Lifts

START: Four-point position

MOVEMENT:

1 Lift one arm forward while extending opposite leg behind you.

2 Keep hips stable and shoulders level throughout.

3 Lower arm and leg back to starting position with control.

4 Alternate sides, completing 10 repetitions per side, 2 sets.

EQUIPMENT
• Mat

FOCUS
• Maintain stable pelvis and keep core engaged
• Keep hips and shoulders level
• Control the movement

Four-Way Ankle (Banded)

EQUIPMENT
- **Chair**
- **Long resistance band**

FOCUS
- Isolate ankle movement
- Maintain leg stability
- Control the movement

START: Sit with band around forefoot, secured in direction opposite to movement.

MOVEMENT:

1 Keep knee and leg stable throughout.

2 Move ankle against band resistance in one direction.

3 Return to starting position with control.

4 Repeat for inward, outward, upward, and downward movements.

5 Complete 10 reps in each direction per side, 1-2 sets.

Front Arm Raises (Weighted)

EQUIPMENT
- **Light weights**

FOCUS
- Maintain neutral spine
- Keep shoulders down
- Control the movement

START: Standing position with weights in hands, palms facing down

MOVEMENT:

1 Engage shoulder blades toward bra line.

2 Lift weights to shoulder height, keeping elbows straight.

3 Keep shoulders down (avoid shrugging).

4 Lower weights with control.

5 Complete 10 repetitions, 1-2 sets.

Front Step Downs

START: Standing position on a low jump box

MOVEMENT:

1 With one leg, reach in front and tap heel on floor next to step.

2 Control movement, keeping hips level and knees properly aligned.

3 Return to starting position with control.

4 Complete 10 repetitions per side, 1-2 sets.

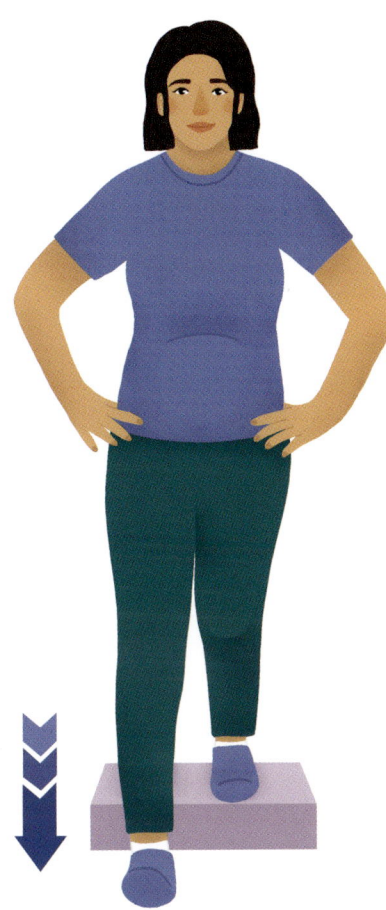

EQUIPMENT
• Low step/box (6 inches)
• Weight (optional)

FOCUS
• Maintain hip stability
• Control the movement
• Keep standing knee aligned

Full Plank

START: Four-point position

MOVEMENT:

1 Extend both legs backward, creating a straight line from head to heels.

2 Engage core and maintain neutral spine.

3 Hold position for 30 seconds.

4 Complete 1-2 sets.

EQUIPMENT
• Mat

FOCUS
• Maintain straight body alignment
• Keep shoulders over wrists
• Engage core throughout

Glute Wall Reach

EQUIPMENT
- Wall

FOCUS
- Maintain balance on standing leg
- Control the reaching movement
- Engage glutes to return

START: Standing position with side toward wall, both knees bent at 30-degree angle

MOVEMENT:

1 Lift outside foot (furthest from wall) a few inches off ground.

2 Reach outside hand across body to touch wall.

3 Reach down and forward along wall.

4 Drive through standing leg glute to return to upright position.

5 Complete 10 repetitions each side, 1-2 sets.

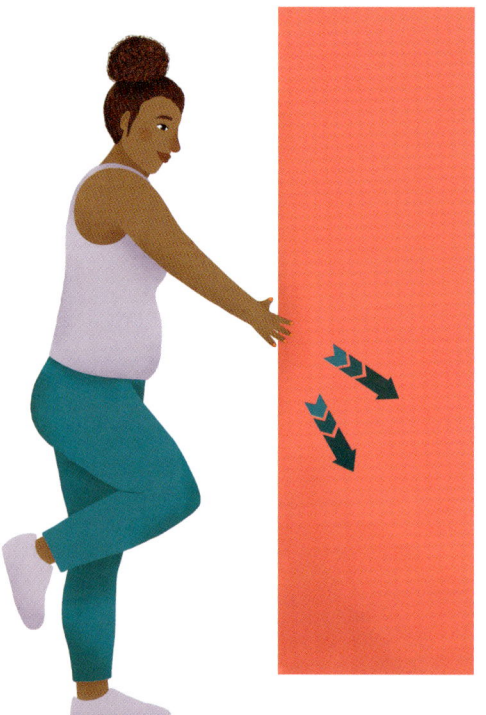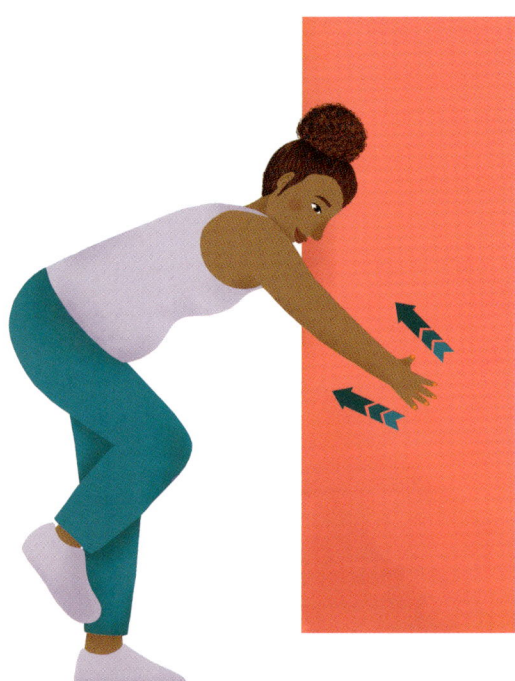

Heel Slides

START: Lying position

MOVEMENT:

1 Slide one heel away from your body until leg is straight.

2 Return to starting position with control, keeping pelvis neutral.

3 Alternate legs, completing 10 repetitions per side, 2 sets.

EQUIPMENT
• Mat

FOCUS
• Keep opposite leg stable
• Maintain neutral pelvis
• Engage core throughout

Hip Thrusters

START: Start with your upper back resting against a bench or jump box, with your hips unsupported

MOVEMENT:

1 Keep feet flat and knees bent at 90-degree angle.

2 Drive hips toward ceiling while maintaining neutral spine.

3 Lower with control to starting position.

4 Complete 10 repetitions, 1-2 sets.

EQUIPMENT
• Bench or jump box

FOCUS
• Maintain neutral spine
• Drive through heels
• Engage core throughout

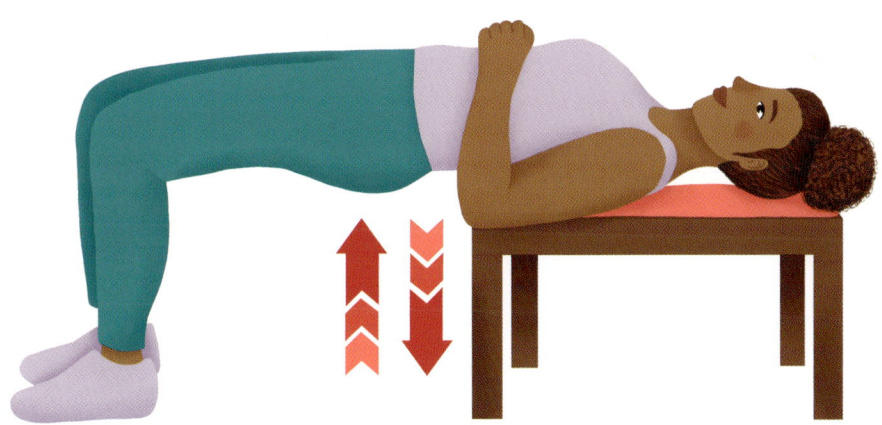

Hops (Banded)

EQUIPMENT
- Loop band
- Agility ladder

Note: If you don't have an agility ladder, mark off a series of spaces that are approximately 15 inches apart.

FOCUS
- Land softly
- Maintain knee alignment and core control
- Control each hop

START: Standing position at beginning of agility ladder with loop band above knees

MOVEMENT:

1 Perform 2 controlled 6-inch hops per box.

2 Maintain knee alignment.

3 Progress through entire ladder.

4 Complete 8 repetitions, 2 sets

Jump Prep

EQUIPMENT
- Loop band

FOCUS
- Maintain knee alignment
- Control the movement
- Keep core engaged

START: Standing position with loop band positioned above knees

MOVEMENT:

1 Lower into shallow squat, keeping knees aligned.

2 Drive hips forward and rise onto toes.

3 Lower heels back to ground with controlled knee alignment.

4 Complete 8 repetitions, 2 sets.

Knee Fall Outs

EQUIPMENT
- Mat

FOCUS
- Keep pelvis stable
- Maintain core engagement
- Control the movement

START: Lying position

MOVEMENT:

1 Lower one knee outward while keeping foot in contact with floor.

2 Return knee to starting position with controlled speed.

3 Alternate sides, completing 10 repetitions per side, 2 sets.

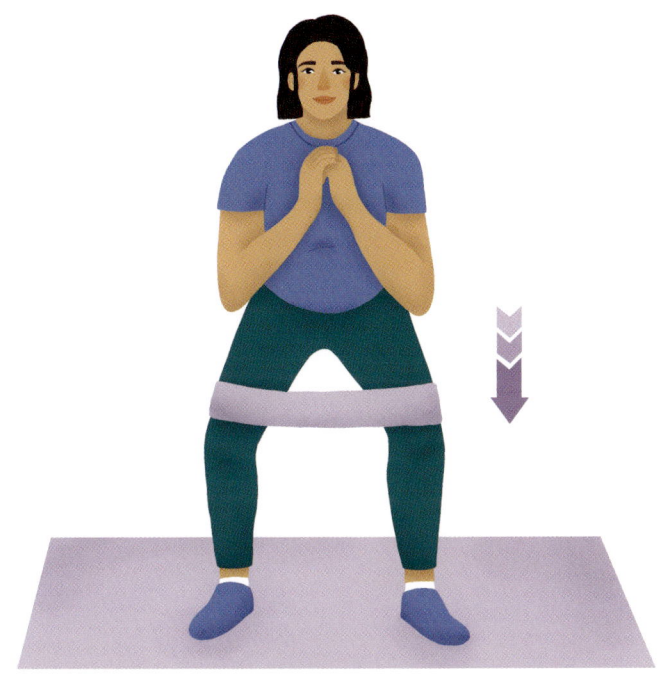

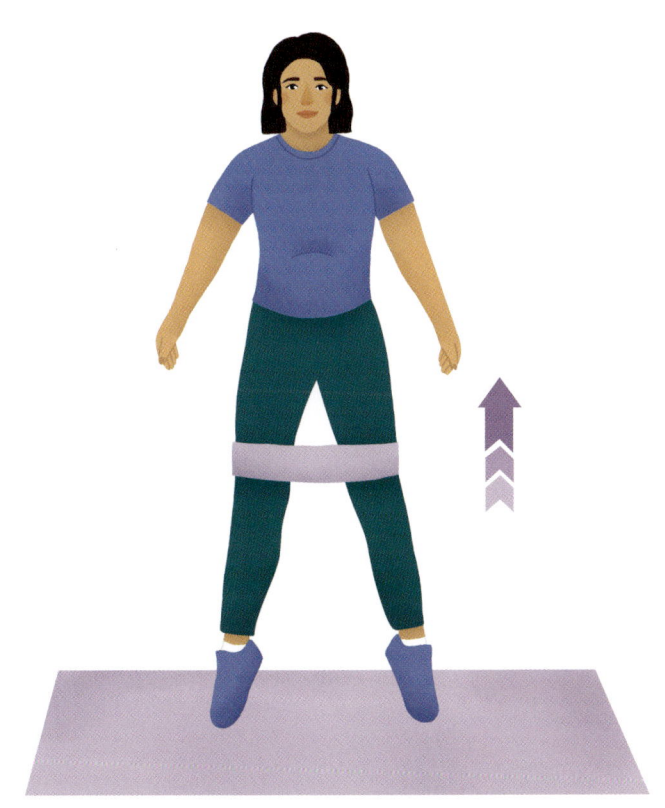

JUMP PREP

Knee Straighteners

EQUIPMENT
• Mat

FOCUS
• Keep pelvis stable
• Maintain level thighs
• Control the movement

START: Lying position

MOVEMENT:

1 Straighten one knee while keeping thighs level with each other.

2 Return to starting position with control, avoiding pelvic movement.

3 Alternate legs, completing 10 repetitions per side, 2 sets.

Kneeling Pallof Press (Banded)

EQUIPMENT
• Long resistance band
• Secure anchor
• Padded surface

FOCUS
• Engage core throughout
• Resist rotation
• Maintain stable pelvis
• Control the movement

START: Standing position with band anchored at your side

MOVEMENT:

1 Hold the other end of the band in both hands at chest level.

2 Step back and lower your back knee onto a padded surface, with your front knee bent at a 90-degree angle.

3 Press your arms straight forward, and maintain tension on the band throughout the movement.

4 Hold briefly then return hands to chest with control.

5 Complete 10 repetitions per side, 1-2 sets.

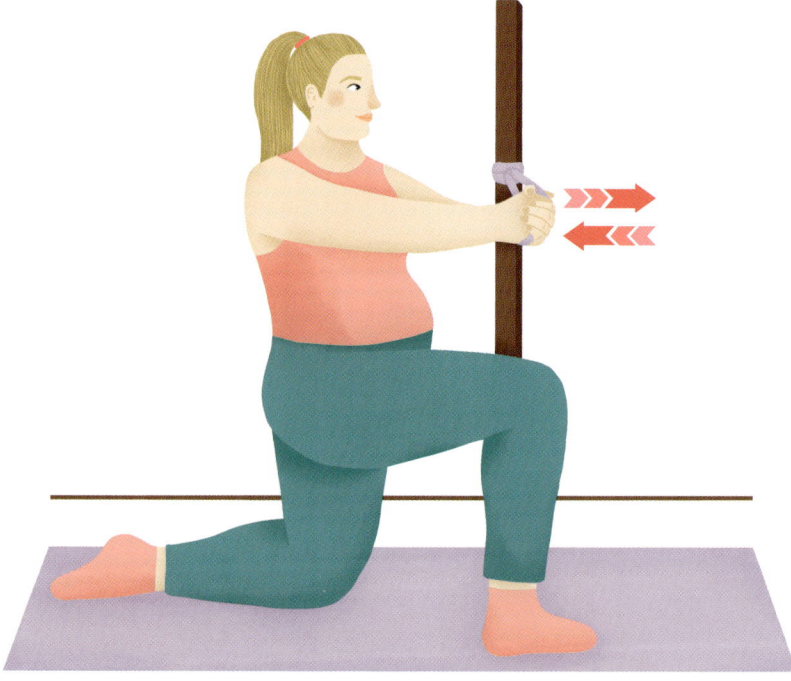

Kneeling Side Plank

START: Kneeling side plank position

MOVEMENT:

1 Ensure hips are stacked and knees bent at 90-degree angle.

2 Hold position for 30 seconds, maintaining proper alignment.

3 Lower with control, then repeat on opposite side.

4 Complete 2 sets per side.

EQUIPMENT
• Mat

FOCUS
• Keep hips aligned and elevated
• Maintain core engagement
• Breathe normally

Kneeling Side Plank Clamshells

START: Kneeling side plank position

MOVEMENT:

1 Ensure hips are stacked with knees bent at 90-degree angle.

2 Keep feet together and rotate top knee toward ceiling.

3 Control the lowering phase as you return to starting position.

4 Complete 10 repetitions per side, 1-2 sets.

EQUIPMENT
• Mat
• Loop band (optional)

FOCUS
• Maintain stable plank position
• Control hip rotation
• Keep core engaged

Kneeling Side Plank Hip Drops

START: Kneeling side plank position

MOVEMENT:

1 Lower hips toward floor with control.

2 Lift hips back up to starting position.

3 Complete 10 repetitions per side, 1-2 sets.

EQUIPMENT
• Mat

FOCUS
• Maintain shoulder stability
• Control the movement
• Maintain core engagement
• Keep body aligned

Kneeling Side Plank Hip Drops with Leg Lift

EQUIPMENT
• Mat
• Loop band (optional)

FOCUS
• Maintain leg lift throughout
• Maintain core engagement
• Control hip movement
• Keep shoulders stable

START: Kneeling side plank position

MOVEMENT:

1 Lift top leg slightly up and backward, engaging glutes.

2 Keep leg elevated throughout the exercise.

3 Lower hips toward floor with control.

4 Lift hips back up to starting position.

5 Complete 10 repetitions per side, 1-2 sets.

Ladder In/Outs

EQUIPMENT
• Agility ladder or marked spaces

FOCUS
• Stay light on feet
• Maintain rhythm
• Keep weight evenly distributed

START: Standing position at beginning of agility ladder

MOVEMENT:

1 Bend your knees into a quarter-squat position, distributing your weight evenly between both feet.

2 Step forward into the first box with your left foot, followed by your right foot (in–in).

3 Using your left foot to step outside the ladder, followed by the right foot (out–out).

4 Continue to the next box, repeat this in–in, out–out pattern as you progress through the ladder.

5 Complete 8 repetitions, 2 sets

Leg Lifts

EQUIPMENT
• Mat

FOCUS
• Keep pelvis stable
• Maintain core engagement
• Control entire movement

START: Lying position

MOVEMENT:

1 Straighten one knee while keeping thighs level.

2 Lower straightened leg toward ground while keeping other leg stable.

3 Lift leg back up to level of opposite thigh without pelvic movement.

4 Bend knee with control to return to starting position.

5 Alternate legs, completing 10 repetitions per side, 2 sets.

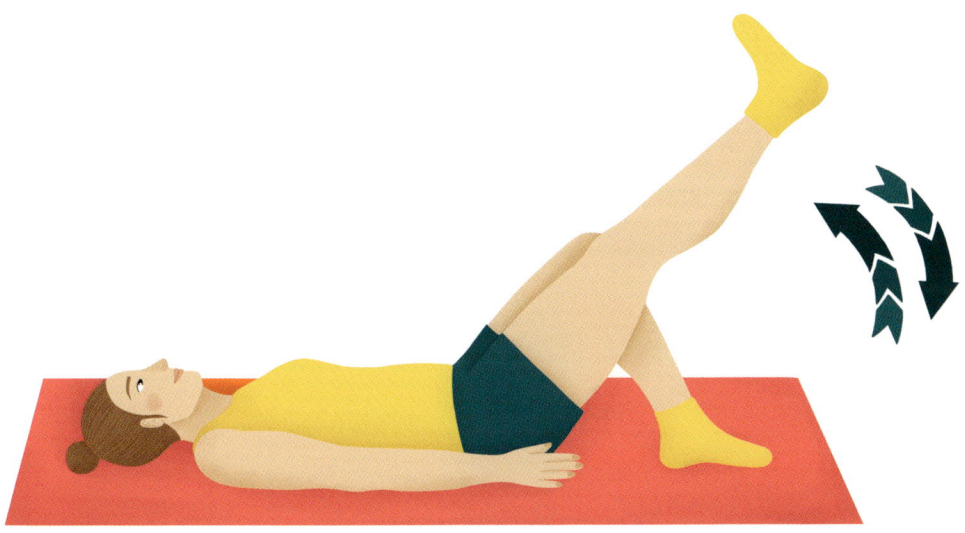

LEG LIFTS

Low Bicycle

START: Lying position, feet lifted with hips and knees at 90-degree angle

MOVEMENT:

1 Extend one leg straight out in front of you.

2 Lower leg only as far as core remains engaged, avoiding back arching.

3 Return to starting position before alternating legs.

4 Complete 10 repetitions per side, 1-2 sets.

EQUIPMENT
• Mat

FOCUS
• Maintain neutral spine
• Keep core engaged
• Control leg movement

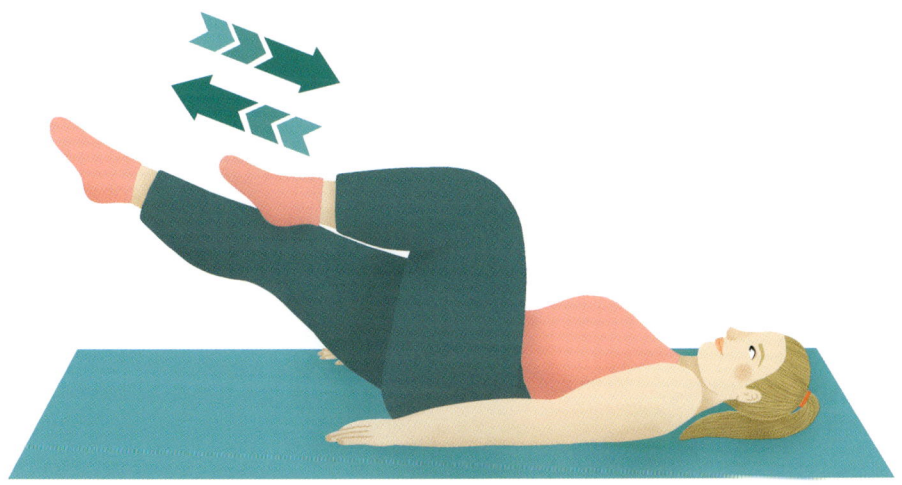

LOW BICYCLE

Marches

EQUIPMENT
• Mat

FOCUS
• Keep pelvis stable
• Avoid rotating hips
• Maintain core engagement

START: Lying position

MOVEMENT:

1 Lift one knee toward chest while keeping other leg stable.

2 Return foot back to ground without side-to-side movement.

3 Alternate legs, completing 10 repetitions per side, 2 sets.

Medium/Full Squats

EQUIPMENT
• Weight (optional)

FOCUS
• Keep knees aligned with toes
• Maintain neutral spine
• Engage core throughout

START: Standing position

MOVEMENT:

1 Lower hips back and down, bending at hips and knees until knees are at 45-degree angle for a medium squat, or a 90-degree angle for a full squat.

2 Distribute weight evenly between heels and balls of feet.

3 Engage glutes to return to standing position, keeping hips slightly tucked.

4 Complete 10 repetitions, 1-2 sets.

Mini Squats

EQUIPMENT
None

FOCUS
• Keep knees aligned with toes
• Distribute weight evenly
• Engage core

START: Standing position

MOVEMENT:

1 Lower hips back and down slightly, bending at knees and hips as if sitting.

2 Distribute weight evenly between heels and balls of feet.

3 Engage glutes to return to standing position, keeping hips slightly tucked.

4 Avoid arching back excessively when standing up.

5 Complete 10 repetitions, 1-2 sets.

Modified Copenhagen on Jump Box

START: Side lying position with top knee supported on raised surface

MOVEMENT:

1 Place forearm slightly under shoulder.

2 Lift hips toward ceiling creating straight line from shoulder to knee.

3 Hold for 30 seconds, keeping hips level without arching back.

4 Complete 1-2 sets per side.

EQUIPMENT
- Jump box or raised surface
- Mat

FOCUS
- Keep spine neutral
- Maintain straight body alignment
- Engage core

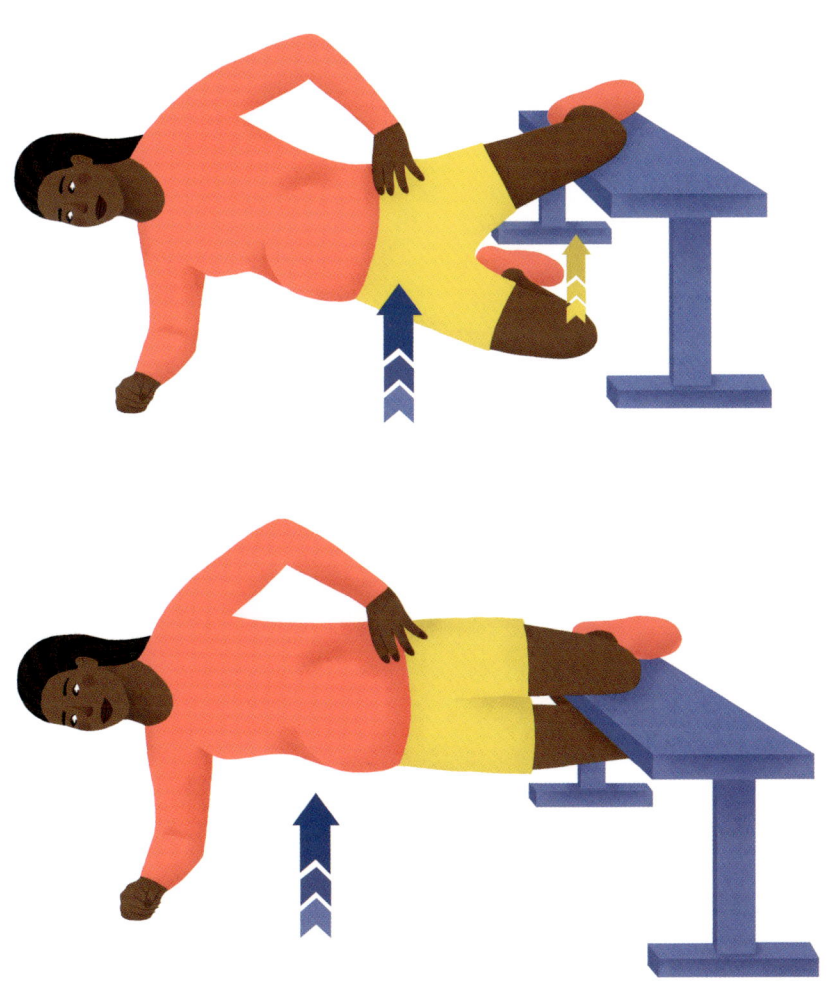

Pull Downs (Banded)

START: Standing position with band secured above, holding ends with equal length in each hand

MOVEMENT:

1. Facing the band, squeeze shoulder blades toward bra line.

2. Pull band down, bending elbows to 90 degrees at shoulder height.

3. Return to starting position with control.

4. Maintain neutral spine throughout.

5. Complete 10 repetitions, 1-2 sets.

Rows (Banded)

START: Standing position with band in both hands, equal length on each side

MOVEMENT:

1. Step back until band has tension when arms are extended.

2. Squeeze shoulder blades together toward bra line.

3. Bend elbows at 90-degree angle, bringing hands toward waist.

4. Return to starting position with control.

5. Complete 10 repetitions, 1-2 sets.

Runner's Balance Challenges

START: Standing position with one knee bent at 30 degrees in mid-stance running position

MOVEMENT:

1. Lift other leg, moving it out to side and slightly back.

2. Keep knee soft on lifted leg.

3. Return to starting position with control.

4. Maintain steady rhythm, as if running.

5. Complete 10 repetitions per side, 1-2 sets.

Runner's Bent-Knee Calf Raises

START: Standing position with knees bent at 30-degree angle

MOVEMENT:

1 Place one foot on chair in front of you with knee bent.

2 Rise onto ball of standing foot, keeping knee bent at 30-degree angle.

3 Hold top position for one second.

4 Lower slowly over 3-second count back to starting position.

5 Complete 20 repetitions per side, 1-2 sets.

EQUIPMENT
- Chair
- Stable surface for support

FOCUS
- Maintain bent knee throughout
- Control the lowering phase
- Keep arch lifted

Runner's Bent-Knee Calf Raises (Weighted)

START: Standing position with knees bent at 30-degree angle

MOVEMENT:

1 Place one foot on chair with knee bent.

2 Hold weight comfortably at side.

3 Rise onto ball of standing foot, keeping knee bent at 30-degree angle.

4 Lower slowly over 3-second count back to starting position.

5 Complete 20 repetitions per side, 1-2 sets.

EQUIPMENT
- Chair
- Weights
- Stable surface

FOCUS
- Maintain control of weight
- Keep knee bent
- Control the movement

Runner's Clamshells

START: Standing position, 2 feet from wall with back toward it

MOVEMENT:

1 Place one foot against the wall behind you.

2 Rotate back knee upward while keeping pelvis stable.

3 Control the movement as you return to starting position.

4 Complete 10 repetitions per side, 1-2 sets.

EQUIPMENT
- Wall

FOCUS
- Keep pelvis stable
- Initiate movement from hip
- Maintain balance

Runner's Clamshells (Banded)

EQUIPMENT
• Wall
• Loop band

FOCUS
• Maintain band tension
• Keep pelvis stable
• Control the movement

START: Standing position, 2 feet from wall with loop band around thighs above knees

MOVEMENT:

1 Place one foot against the wall behind you and bend the standing leg to 30-degrees.

2 Rotate back knee upward against band resistance while keeping pelvis stable.

3 Control the movement as you return to starting position.

4 Complete 10 repetitions per side, 1-2 sets.

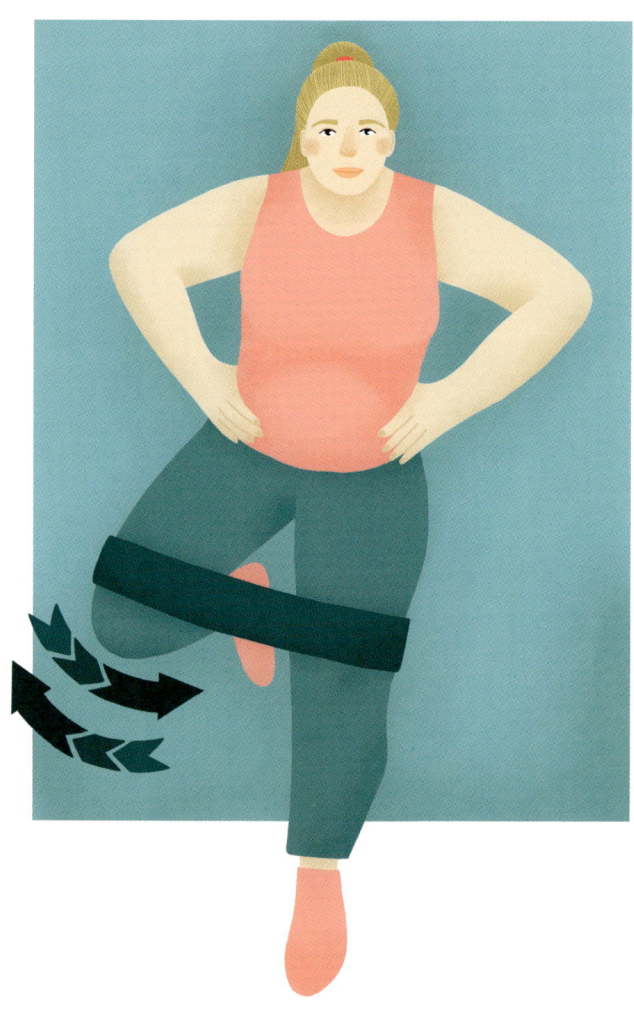

Runner's Toe Taps

START: Lying position, feet lifted with hips at 90-degree and knees at 30-degree angle

MOVEMENT:

1 Lower one heel toward floor keeping knee bent at 30-degree angle.

2 Keep opposite leg stable in starting position.

3 Touch ground lightly with heel then return to starting position.

4 Alternate legs, completing 10 repetitions per side, 1–2 sets.

EQUIPMENT
• Mat

FOCUS
• Maintain 30-degree knee bend
• Keep core engaged
• Control the movement

Scalene Stretch

START: Seated position

MOVEMENT:

1 Place fingers over opposite side collarbone.

2 Put other hand on top of fingers.

3 Tip head to side (away from hands) and back.

4 Gently press on collarbone to deepen stretch.

5 Drop shoulder down with each exhale.

6 Hold for 30 seconds per side, 1–2 sets.

EQUIPMENT
• Chair

FOCUS
• Keep shoulder relaxed
• Breathe into the stretch
• Feel release in neck

Scissor Jumps

START: Standing position

MOVEMENT:

1 Step forward with one foot, keeping your feet hip-width apart.

2 Bend both knees until your front knee forms a 45-degree angle.

3 Jump and switch legs in midair, keeping your knees aligned over your ankles.

4 Land softly in the lunge position, with the other leg now pointing forward, ensuring your front knee is aligned over your ankle.

5 Complete 8 repetitions, 2 sets.

EQUIPMENT
None

FOCUS
• Land softly
• Maintain knee alignment
• Keep neutral pelvis

Seated Hip Abduction

EQUIPMENT
- Chair

FOCUS
- Keep spine neutral
- Feel outer hip engagement
- Control the movement

START: Seated position

MOVEMENT:

1 Press knees outward while keeping feet flat on floor.

2 Control movement as you return to starting position.

3 Maintain proper rib cage and pelvis alignment throughout.

4 Complete 10 repetitions, 1-2 sets.

Seated Hip Abduction (Banded)

EQUIPMENT
- Chair
- Loop band

FOCUS
- Maintain band tension
- Keep spine neutral
- Control the movement

START: Seated position with loop band around thighs just above knees

MOVEMENT:

1 Press knees outward against band resistance.

2 Control movement as you return to starting position.

3 Maintain proper rib cage and pelvis alignment throughout.

4 Complete 10 repetitions, 1-2 sets.

Seated Hip Adduction

EQUIPMENT
- Chair
- Pillow/ball (optional)

FOCUS
- Maintain upright posture
- Feel inner thigh engagement
- Control the movement

START: Seated position with feet flat on floor, hip-width apart

MOVEMENT:

1 Press knees together with controlled pressure. Optional: Use a pillow or ball between your knees for muscle feedback or added comfort.

2 Hold for 5 seconds.

3 Release with control.

4 Complete 10 repetitions, 1-2 sets.

Seated Leg Curls (Banded)

START: Seated position with loop band around ankles

MOVEMENT:

1 Place one foot firmly on chair seat with toes pointing forward.

2 Pull other leg backward while keeping thighs parallel.

3 Return to starting position slowly, maintaining band tension.

4 Complete 10 repetitions per side, 1-2 sets.

EQUIPMENT
- **Two chairs**
- **Loop band**

FOCUS
- Keep thighs parallel
- Maintain upright posture
- Control the movement

Seated Leg Extensions (Banded)

START: Seated position with loop band around ankles

MOVEMENT:

1 Place feet flat on floor, hip-width apart.

2 Straighten one leg with control, keeping thighs parallel.

3 Return to starting position slowly, maintaining band tension.

4 Complete 10 repetitions per side, 1-2 sets.

EQUIPMENT
- **Chair**
- **Loop band**

FOCUS
- Keep thighs parallel
- Maintain upright posture
- Control the movement

Seated Marches

START: Seated position

MOVEMENT:

1 Slightly lean forward, maintaining straight back.

2 Engage hip into socket and lift one knee toward ceiling.

3 Control descent without shifting weight to opposite hip.

4 Alternate legs, completing 10 repetitions per side, 1-2 sets.

EQUIPMENT
- **Chair**

FOCUS
- Maintain tall posture
- Keep hips level
- Control the movement

Seated Marches (Banded)

EQUIPMENT
• Chair
• Loop band

FOCUS
• Maintain band tension throughout
• Keep hips level
• Control the movement

START: Seated position at edge of chair with loop band around feet in figure-eight shape

MOVEMENT:

1 Slightly lean forward, maintaining straight back.

2 Engage hip into socket and lift one knee toward ceiling against band resistance.

3 Control descent without shifting weight to opposite hip.

4 Alternate legs, completing 10 repetitions per side, 1-2 sets.

Seated Pelvic Tilts on Ball

EQUIPMENT
• Therapy/stability ball

FOCUS
• Isolate movement to lower back
• Keep upper back stable
• Move with control

START: Seated position on a therapy ball

MOVEMENT:

1 Arch lower back toward belly, lifting tailbone.

2 Pause, then slowly tuck tailbone under while rounding lower back.

3 Keep upper back stable throughout the movement.

4 Complete 10 repetitions, 2 sets.

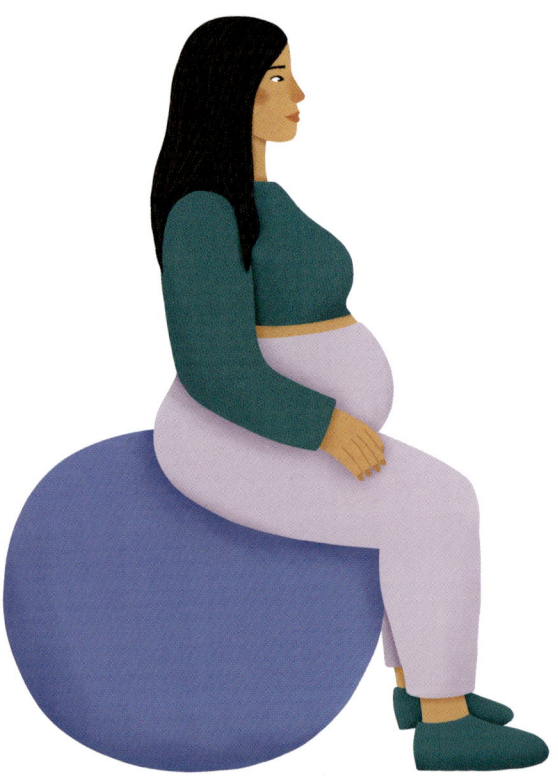

Seated Shoulder Press (Weighted)

START: Seated position with weights at shoulder height, palms forward, elbows at 90 degrees

MOVEMENT:

1 Press weights overhead while maintaining neutral spine.

2 Keep shoulders down (avoid shrugging).

3 Lower weights with control to starting position.

4 Complete 10 repetitions, 1-2 sets.

EQUIPMENT
• Chair
• Light weights

FOCUS
• Maintain neutral spine
• Control the movement

Seated Twist Stretch

START: Seated position

MOVEMENT:

1 Place one hand on outside of opposite knee, other arm across chair back.

2 Inhale, expanding sides of ribs.

3 Exhale, drawing sternum toward belly button.

4 Rotate from belly button toward hand on knee, deepening with each exhale.

5 Hold for 30 seconds per side, 1-2 sets.

EQUIPMENT
• Chair

FOCUS
• Initiate twist from core
• Keep spine tall
• Breathe into the stretch

Side-Lying Clamshells

START: Side-lying position

MOVEMENT:

1 Gently engage top hip back into socket.

2 Keep feet together and rotate top knee toward ceiling.

3 Control the lowering phase as you return to starting position.

4 Complete 10 repetitions per side, 1-2 sets.

EQUIPMENT
• Mat

FOCUS
• Keep pelvis stable
• Initiate movement from hip
• Maintain feet contact

Side-Lying Clamshells (Banded)

EQUIPMENT
• Mat
• Loop band

FOCUS
• Maintain band tension
• Keep pelvis stable
• Control the movement

START: Side-lying position with loop band around thighs above knees, hips stacked

MOVEMENT:

1 Gently engage top hip back into socket.

2 Keep feet together and rotate top knee toward ceiling against band resistance.

3 Control the lowering phase as you return to starting position.

4 Complete 10 repetitions per side, 1-2 sets.

Side-Lying Hip Abduction

EQUIPMENT
• Mat

FOCUS
• Initiate movement from glutes
• Prevent back arching
• Control the movement

START: Side-lying position with bottom leg bent for support, top leg straight

MOVEMENT:

1 Lift top leg to side and slightly back, engaging glutes.

2 Keep low back from arching during movement.

3 Lower leg halfway down with control.

4 Complete 10 repetitions per side, 1-2 sets.

Side-Lying Hip Abduction (Banded)

EQUIPMENT
• Mat
• Loop band

FOCUS
• Maintain band tension
• Prevent back arching
• Control the movement

START: Side-lying position with bottom leg bent for support, top leg straight, with loop band around thighs just above knees

MOVEMENT:

1 Bend bottom leg for support, keep top leg straight.

2 Lift top leg against band resistance, engaging glutes.

3 Lower leg halfway down with control.

4 Complete 10 repetitions per side, 1-2 sets.

Side-Lying Rotation Stretch

START: Side-lying position with bottom leg straight, top leg bent with foot in bottom knee crease

MOVEMENT:

1 Place bottom hand on top knee.

2 Raise top arm toward ceiling in Y position.

3 Follow hand with eyes as you rotate toward ceiling from bra line.

4 Hold for 30 seconds, deepening rotation with each exhale.

5 Complete 1-2 sets per side.

EQUIPMENT
• Mat
• Pillow (optional)

FOCUS
• Initiate rotation from upper back
• Keep hips stacked
• Breathe into the stretch

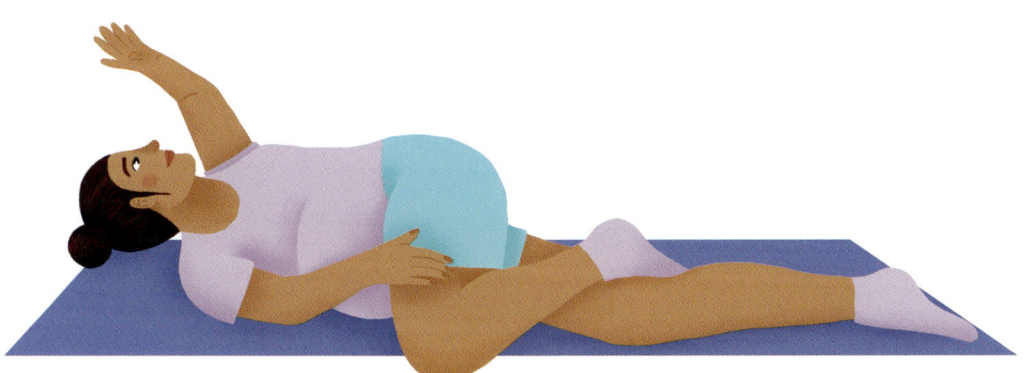

Side Lunges

EQUIPMENT
• Weights (optional)

FOCUS
• Keep toes pointing forward
• Sit back into hip
• Engage glutes to return

START: Standing position

MOVEMENT:

1 Step out to one side, keeping toes pointing forward.

2 Bend the stepping leg at hip and knee while keeping other leg straight.

3 Engage glutes to return to starting position.

4 Complete 10 repetitions per side, 1–2 sets.

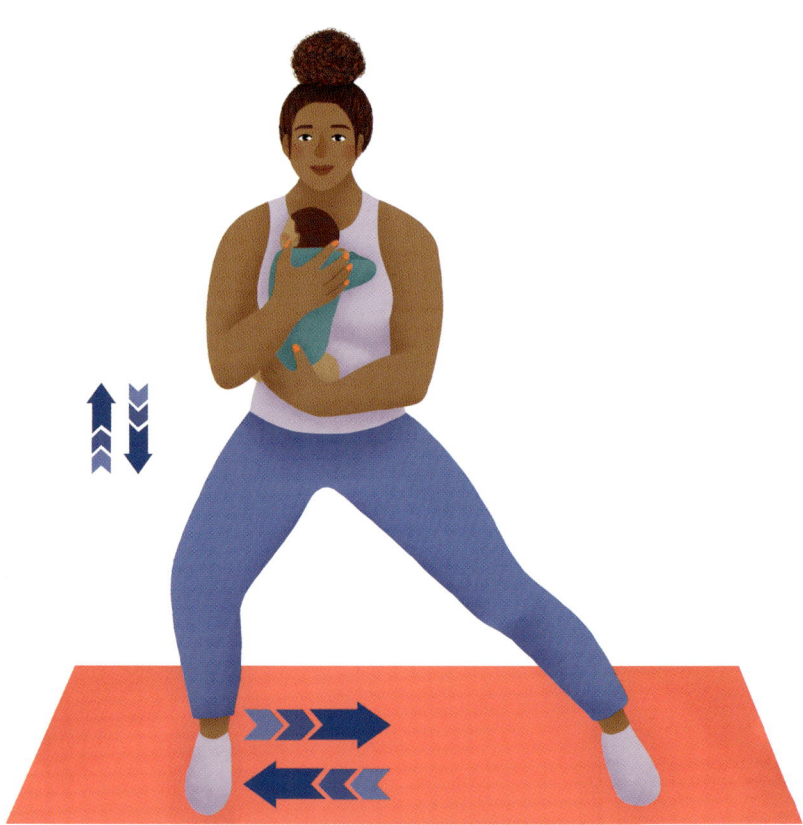

Side Plank

START: Side plank position

MOVEMENT:

1 Ensure hips and feet are stacked with straight body alignment.

2 Hold position for 30 seconds, maintaining proper form.

3 Lower with control, then repeat on opposite side.

4 Complete 2 sets per side.

EQUIPMENT
• Mat

FOCUS
• Maintain straight body alignment
• Keep hips elevated
• Engage core throughout

Side Plank Hip Drops

START: Side plank position

MOVEMENT:

1 Lower hips toward floor with control.

2 Lift hips back up to starting position.

3 Complete 10 repetitions per side, 1-2 sets.

EQUIPMENT
• Mat

FOCUS
• Maintain body alignment
• Control the movement
• Keep shoulders stable
• Engage core throughout

Side Plank Leg Lifts

START: Side plank or kneeling side plank position

MOVEMENT:

1 Lift top leg slightly up and backward, focusing on glute engagement.

2 Hold for 1 second at peak position.

3 Lower leg to starting position and hold for 1 second.

4 Complete 10 repetitions per side, 1-2 sets.

EQUIPMENT
• Mat
• Loop band (optional)

FOCUS
• Maintain stable plank position
• Keep hips stacked
• Engage glutes during lift
• Engage core throughout

Side Step Downs

EQUIPMENT
- Low step/box
  (6 inches)
- Weights (optional)

FOCUS
- Maintain hip stability
- Control the movement
- Keep standing knee aligned

START: Standing position on a low jump box

MOVEMENT:

1 With one leg, reach to your side and tap heel on floor next to the step or jump box.

2 Control movement, keeping hips level and knees properly aligned.

3 Return to starting position with control.

4 Complete 10 repetitions per side, 1–2 sets.

Side Steps

EQUIPMENT
None

FOCUS
- Keep hips level
- Maintain knee alignment
- Control lateral movement

START: Standing position

MOVEMENT:

1 Bend knees into mini squat position, engaging core.

2 Step sideways while keeping hips level.

3 Control the movement, ensuring toes remain pointing forward.

4 Keep knees aligned over toes throughout movement.

5 Complete 10 repetitions in each direction, 1–2 sets.

Side Steps (Banded)

EQUIPMENT
- Loop band

FOCUS
- Maintain band tension
- Keep hips level
- Control lateral movement

START: Standing position with loop band around thighs above knees or at ankles

MOVEMENT:

1 Bend knees into mini squat position, engaging core.

2 Step sideways against band resistance while keeping hips level.

3 Control the movement, ensuring toes remain pointing forward.

4 Keep knees aligned over toes throughout movement.

5 Complete 10 repetitions in each direction, 1–2 sets.

Single-Leg Balance

START: Standing position

MOVEMENT:

1 Lift one leg off ground while keeping hips level.

2 Maintain balance for 30 seconds, using minimal support if needed.

3 Complete 2 repetitions per side, 1-2 sets.

EQUIPMENT
• Stable surface for support

FOCUS
• Keep hips level
• Engage core
• Maintain upright posture

Single-Leg Balance Clock Reaches

START: Standing position with one leg lifted off ground

MOVEMENT:

1 Tap free heel to different points around an imaginary clock (one full rotation equals one repetition).

2 Reach as far as balance allows while maintaining stability.

3 Keep hips and knees aligned throughout movement

4 Complete 5 repetitions per side, 1-2 sets.

EQUIPMENT
None

FOCUS
• Maintain balance
• Control reaches
• Keep supporting knee aligned

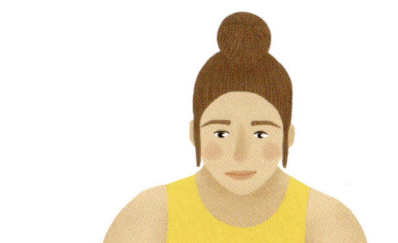

Single-Leg Bridges

EQUIPMENT
• Mat

FOCUS
• Maintain level hips
• Control the movement
• Avoid arching back

START: Lying position

MOVEMENT:

1 Draw one bent knee toward chest, keeping angle greater than 90 degrees.

2 Press through grounded foot to lift hips.

3 Keep hips level as you lower pelvis back down with control.

4 Complete 10 repetitions per side, 1-2 sets.

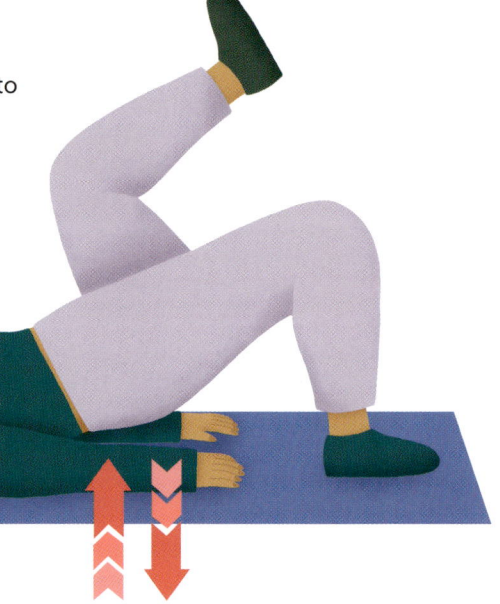

Single-Leg Bridges (Weighted)

EQUIPMENT
• Weight

FOCUS
• Maintain level hips
• Control the weight
• Engage working leg

START: Lying position with weight placed across one upper thigh

MOVEMENT:

1 Using the weighted leg as your working leg, draw opposite knee toward chest, keeping angle greater than 90 degrees.

2 Press through weighted leg to lift hips.

3 Keep hips level as you lower pelvis back down with control.

4 Complete 10 repetitions per side, 1-2 sets.

Single-Leg Calf Raises

START: Standing position near stable surface

MOVEMENT:

1 Shift all your weight onto one leg, then lift non-working leg off ground.

2 Rise onto ball of working foot.

3 Hold for one second at top position.

4 Lower with control back to starting position.

5 Complete 10 repetitions per side, 1-2 sets.

EQUIPMENT
• Stable surface for support
• Weights (optional)

FOCUS
• Maintain balance throughout
• Control the movement
• Keep arch lifted

Single-Leg Hops (Forward/Backward)

START: Standing position in back corner of target square, balancing on one leg

MOVEMENT:

1 Hop forward over the line, landing softly on ball of foot.

2 Hop straight back while maintaining control.

3 Keep movements quick and light, staying close to the line.

4 Complete 8 repetitions per leg, 2 sets.

EQUIPMENT
• Target square (tape or markers)

FOCUS
• Land softly with bent knee
• Maintain balance
• Control each landing

Single-Leg Hops (Side-to-Side)

START: Standing position in back corner of target square, balancing on one leg

MOVEMENT:

1 Hop sideways over the line, landing softly on ball of foot.

2 Return to starting position immediately while maintaining control.

3 Keep movements quick and light, staying close to the line.

4 Complete 8 repetitions per leg, 2 sets.

EQUIPMENT
• Target square (tape or markers)

FOCUS
• Land softly with bent knee
• Maintain balance
• Control each landing

Single-Leg Squats

EQUIPMENT
- Weights (optional)

FOCUS
- Keep supporting knee aligned with foot
- Maintain balance
- Control the movement

START: Standing position

MOVEMENT:

1 Lift one leg, bringing hip and knee to 90-degree angle.

2 Lower into mini squat position on supporting leg.

3 Return to starting position with control.

4 Complete 10 repetitions per side, 1-2 sets.

Single-Leg Squats at a Wall

EQUIPMENT
- Wall

FOCUS
- Keep supporting knee aligned with foot
- Use wall for minimal support
- Maintain balanced posture

START: Standing position parallel to wall with inside leg closest to wall

MOVEMENT:

1 Lift inside leg, bringing hip and knee to 90-degree angle.

2 Gently press knee of inside leg into wall for stability.

3 Lower into mini squat position on supporting leg.

4 Return to starting position with control.

5 Complete 10 repetitions per side, 1-2 sets.

Single-Leg Squats to Runner's Drive

EQUIPMENT
- Weights (optional)

FOCUS
- Coordinate arm and leg movements to mimic running
- Maintain balance
- Control the movement

START: Standing position

MOVEMENT:

1 Lift one leg, bringing hip and knee to 90-degree angle.

2 Lower into mini squat position on supporting leg.

3 While returning to standing position, drive opposite arm forward.

4 Bend elbow and shoulder at 90-degree angle in running form.

5 Complete 10 repetitions per side, 1-2 sets.

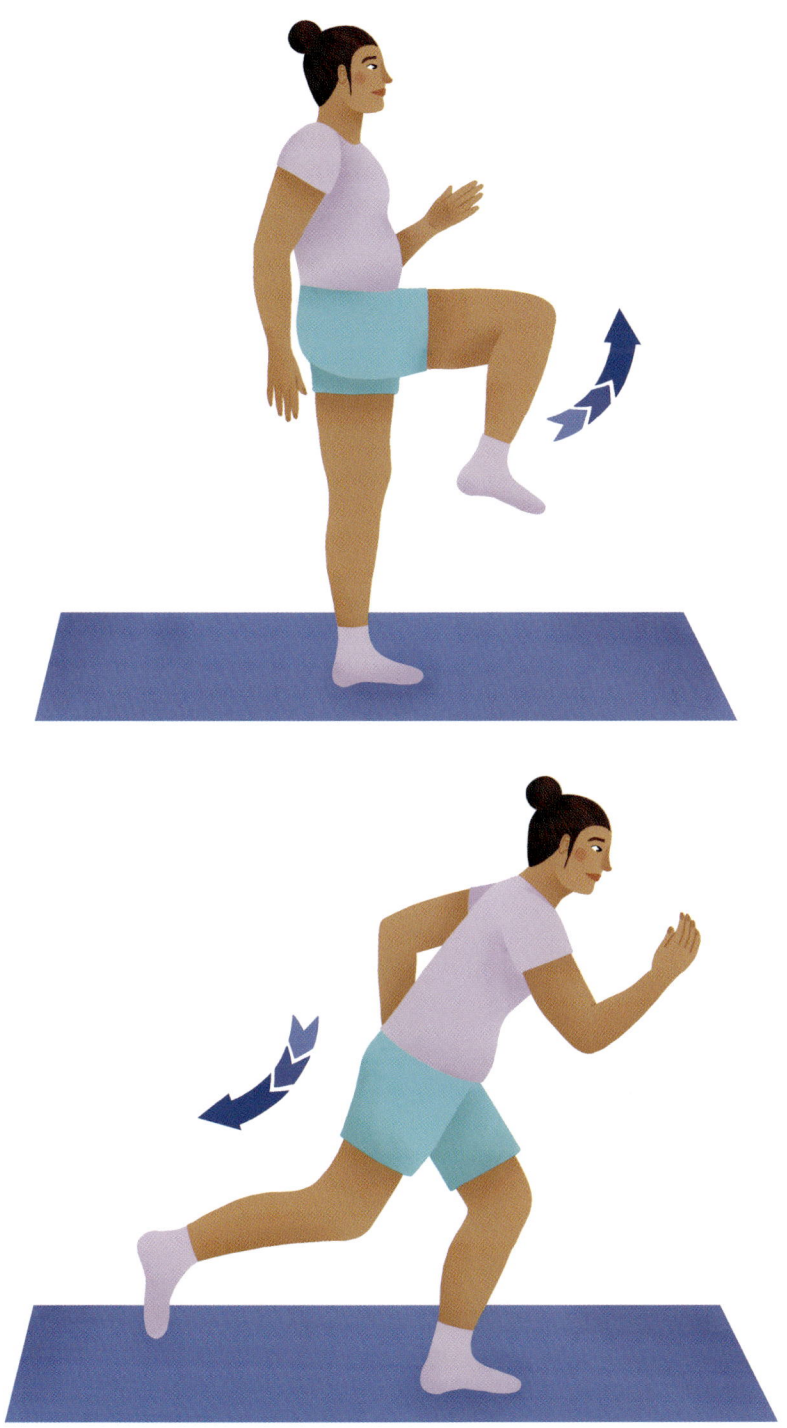

SINGLE-LEG SQUATS TO RUNNER'S DRIVE

Single-Leg to Single-Arm Row (Banded)

EQUIPMENT
- Long resistance band
- Secure anchor

FOCUS
- Coordinate arm and leg movement
- Maintain balance
- Control the movement

START: Standing position on one leg, holding band in opposite-side hand

MOVEMENT:

1. Lift non-working leg to hip height, knee bent.

2. Hinge forward, extending leg back until parallel to ground.

3. Perform rowing motion, pulling elbow back at 90 degrees.

4. Return to standing by engaging standing-leg glute.

5. Complete 10 repetitions per side, 1-2 sets.

Sit to Stand

EQUIPMENT
- Chair

FOCUS
- Keep knees aligned with second toes
- Distribute weight evenly across both feet
- Engage core

START: Seated position with feet slightly tucked under knees

MOVEMENT:

1. Lean forward, bringing your nose over your toes.

2. Press through feet evenly as you stand up.

3. Control your descent as you return to seated position.

4. Repeat for 10 repetitions, 2 sets.

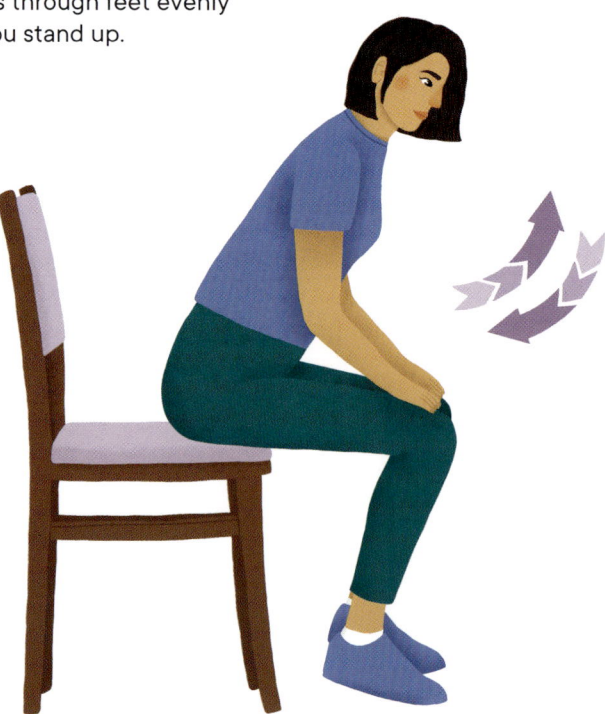

Split-Stance Romanian Deadlifts

START: Standing position with one foot 1.5 feet behind you, ball of foot on floor

MOVEMENT:

1 Center your weight on front leg.

2 Hold a weight in opposite hand.

3 Hinge forward at hips, keeping back flat.

4 Tuck pelvis slightly as you rise.

5 Engage glutes to drive hips forward.

6 Complete 10 repetitions per side, 1–2 sets.

EQUIPMENT
- **Weight (optional)**

FOCUS
- Keep back flat
- Hinge from hips
- Engage glutes to return

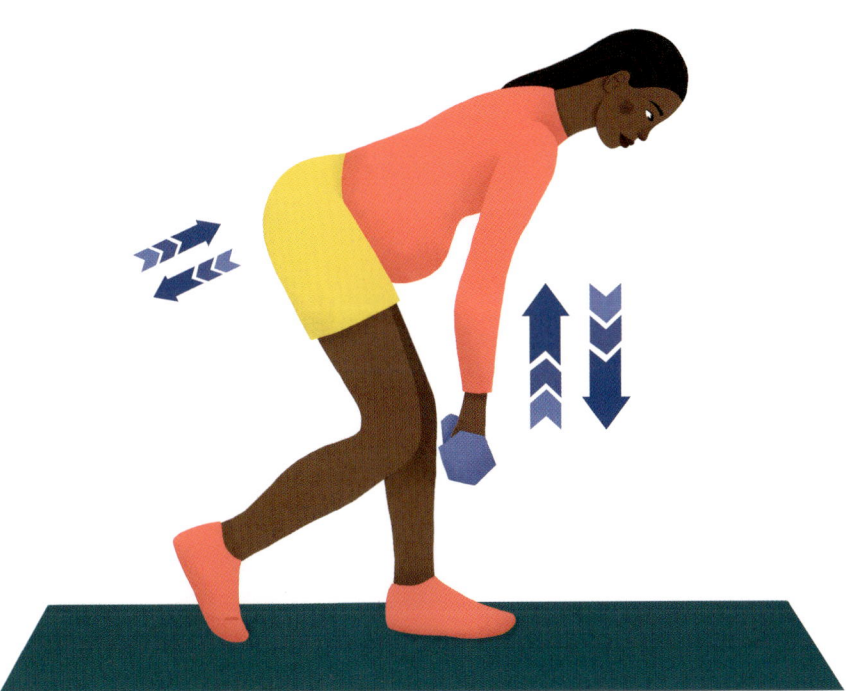

Split-Stance Row (Banded)

START: Standing position with band in hand opposite to forward foot

MOVEMENT:

1 Position back foot about 1.5 feet behind front foot.

2 Squeeze shoulder blade toward bra line.

3 Bend elbow at 90-degree angle, bringing hand toward waist.

4 Return to starting position with control.

5 Complete 10 repetitions per side, 1-2 sets.

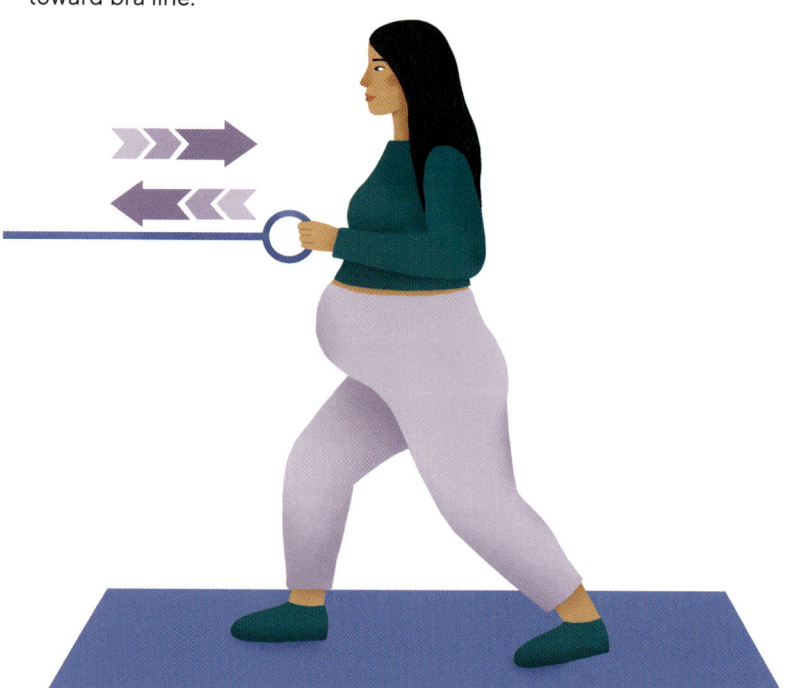

Standing Hip Abduction

START: Standing position, holding onto stable surface for support

MOVEMENT:

1 Lift one leg to side and slightly back, focusing on glute engagement.

2 Return to starting position with control.

3 Complete 10 repetitions per side, 1-2 sets.

Standing Hip Abduction (Banded)

START: Standing position with resistance band secured to door, looped above knee or around ankle

MOVEMENT:

1 Position with band pulling leg toward midline.

2 Move leg away from midline against band resistance.

3 Return to starting position with control.

4 Complete 10 repetitions per side, 1-2 sets.

EQUIPMENT
- Long resistance band
- Door anchor

FOCUS
- Maintain resistance throughout
- Keep hips level
- Control the movement

Standing Hip Adduction

START: Standing position, holding onto stable surface for support

MOVEMENT:

1 Cross your leg in front of you with control.

2 Return to starting position.

3 Cross your leg behind you with control.

4 Return to starting position.

5 Complete 10 repetitions per side, 1-2 sets.

EQUIPMENT
- Stable surface for support

FOCUS
- Keep hips level
- Control the movement
- Maintain balance

Standing Hip Adduction (Banded)

START: Standing position with resistance band secured to door, looped above knee or around ankle

MOVEMENT:

1 Position on outside leg with band creating resistance away from midline.

2 Move leg across midline against band resistance in front or behind you.

3 Return to starting position with control.

4 Complete 10 repetitions per side, 1-2 sets.

EQUIPMENT
- Long resistance band
- Door anchor

FOCUS
- Maintain resistance throughout
- Keep hips level
- Control the movement

Standing Hip Flexor Stretch

EQUIPMENT
Wall

FOCUS
• Keep torso upright
• Engage glutes
• Feel stretch in
  front hip

START: Standing position

MOVEMENT:

1 Step back with one foot, keeping your feet hip-width apart.

2 Lower hips by bending front
   knee, then activate glutes to
   push hips forward until stretch
   felt in front of hip.

3 Hold for 30 seconds, ensuring
   hips face forward throughout.

4 Complete 1-2 sets per side.

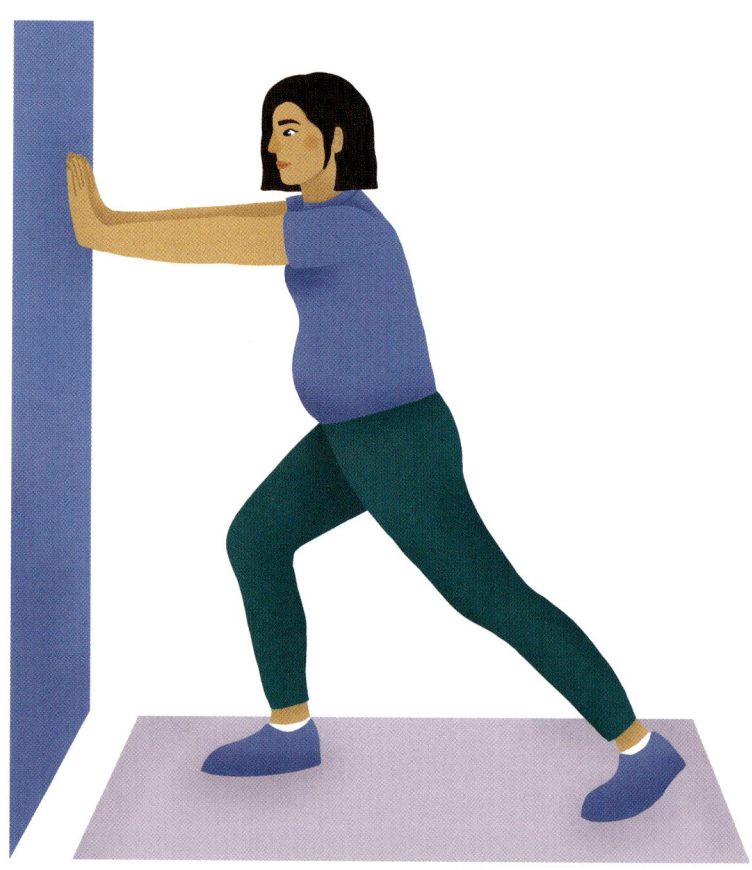

Standing Quadricep Stretch

START: Standing position with stable surface behind you for support

MOVEMENT:

1 Reach back with one leg to rest ankle on surface.

2 Lower hips by bending front knee.

3 Activate glutes to push hips forward until stretch felt in front of thigh.

4 Hold for 30 seconds, ensuring hips face forward throughout.

5 Complete 1-2 sets per side.

EQUIPMENT
- **Two chairs or stable surfaces**

FOCUS
- Keep torso upright
- Maintain balance
- Adjust height as needed

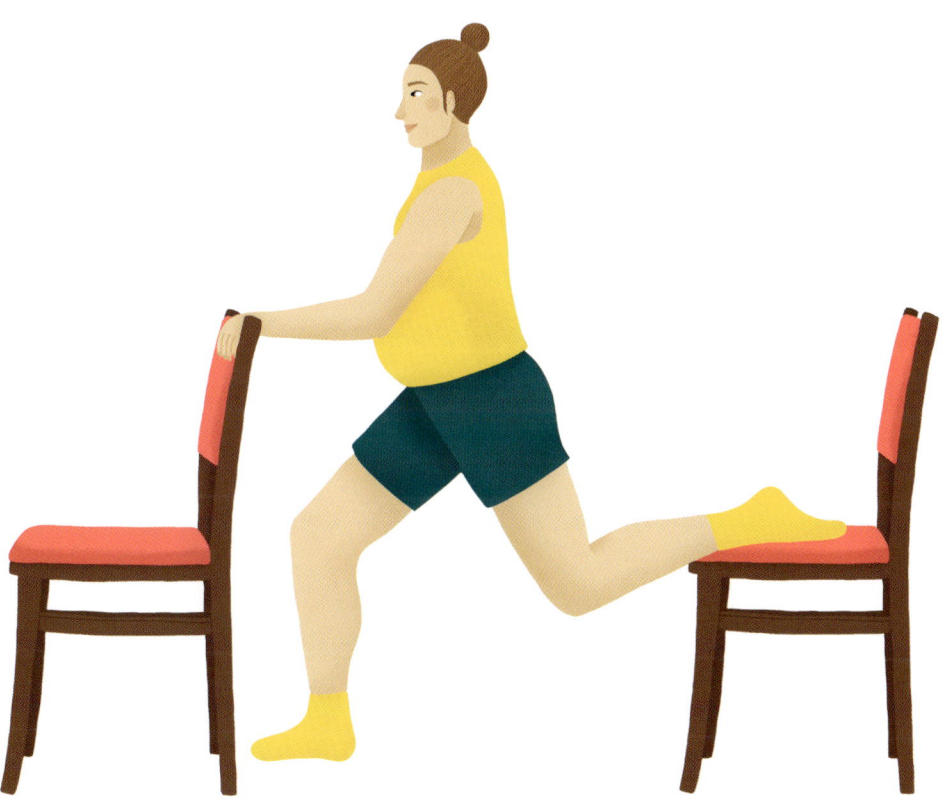

Standing Snow Angels

EQUIPMENT
• Wall

FOCUS
• Keep ribs down
• Maintain wall contact
• Focus on shoulder blade movement

START: Standing position with back flat against wall, knees slightly bent

MOVEMENT:

1 Position arms at shoulder height, elbows bent at 90-degree angle.

2 Keep wrists and elbows in contact with wall, ribs pulled down.

3 Slide arms up toward ceiling, crossing wrists at top.

4 Lower arms with control, maintaining wall contact.

5 Complete 10 repetitions, 1-2 sets.

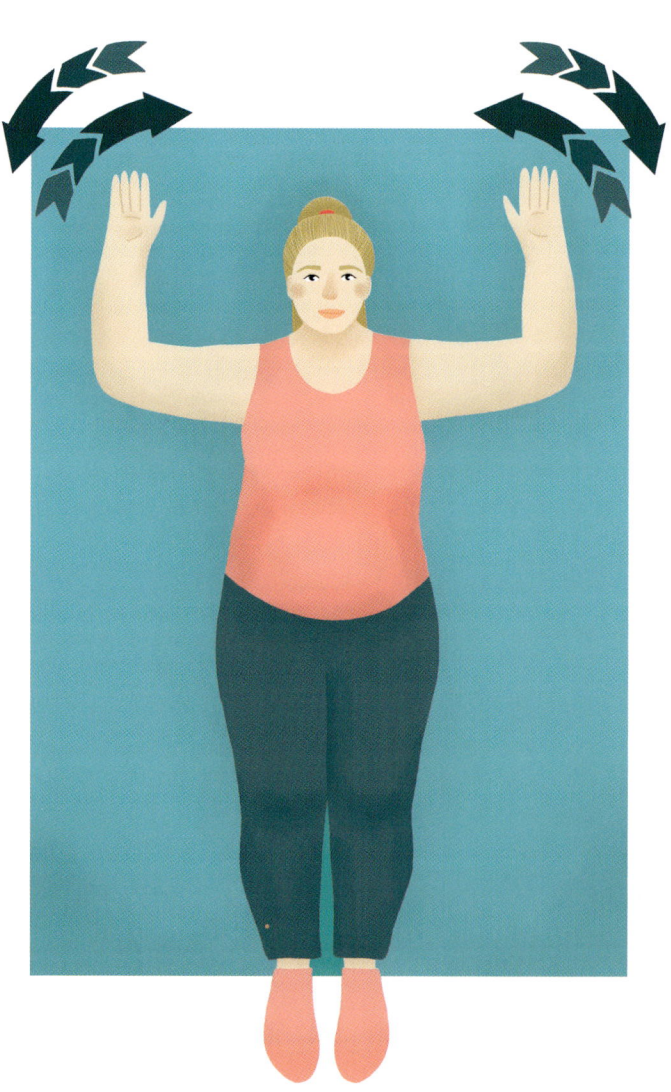

Thread Needle Stretch

START: Four-point position

MOVEMENT:

1 Slide one hand between opposite hand and knee, palm facing up.

2 Gently rest shoulder and side of head on floor.

3 Breathe into ribs, deepening stretch with each exhale.

4 Hold for 30 seconds, avoiding weight on head.

5 Complete 1-2 sets per side.

EQUIPMENT
• Mat

FOCUS
• Keep weight off head
• Breathe into rib cage
• Feel rotation in upper back

Toe Taps

START: Lying position

MOVEMENT:

1 Lift your feet, positioning your hips and knees at a 90-degree angle.

2 Lower one heel toward floor while keeping knee bent at 90-degree angle.

3 Keep opposite leg stable in starting position.

4 Touch ground lightly with heel then return to starting position.

5 Alternate legs, completing 10 repetitions per side, 1-2 sets.

EQUIPMENT
None

FOCUS
• Maintain 90-degree knee bend
• Keep core engaged
• Control the movement

Triceps (Banded)

START: Standing position, facing away from anchor with band ends in each hand

MOVEMENT:

1 Position elbows at sides, bent at 90-degree angle.

2 Straighten arms against band resistance.

3 Keep upper arms still throughout movement.

4 Return to starting position with control.

5 Complete 10 repetitions, 1-2 sets.

EQUIPMENT
• Long resistance band
• Secure anchor

FOCUS
• Keep elbows close to body
• Isolate triceps
• Control the movement

Wall Copenhagen with Runner's Drive

EQUIPMENT
- Wall

FOCUS
- Keep pelvis level
- Control leg movement
- Maintain core engagement

START: Standing position with side facing wall at 2–3 feet distance

MOVEMENT:

1 Place forearm on wall at shoulder height.

2 Lift inside knee (closest to wall) to hip height without tilting pelvis.

3 Straighten leg and extend it behind you.

4 Return knee to hip height in front of you.

5 Complete 10 repetitions per side, 1–2 sets.

Wall Push-Up Plus

EQUIPMENT
- Wall

FOCUS
- Control shoulder blade movement
- Maintain alignment
- Keep core engaged

START: Standing position 12–16 inches from wall with hands at shoulder height

MOVEMENT:

1 Engage shoulder blades by pushing chest slightly backward.

2 Lower chest toward wall, performing push-up motion.

3 Push back to starting position.

4 Maintain slight backward chest position throughout.

5 Complete 10 repetitions, 1–2 sets.

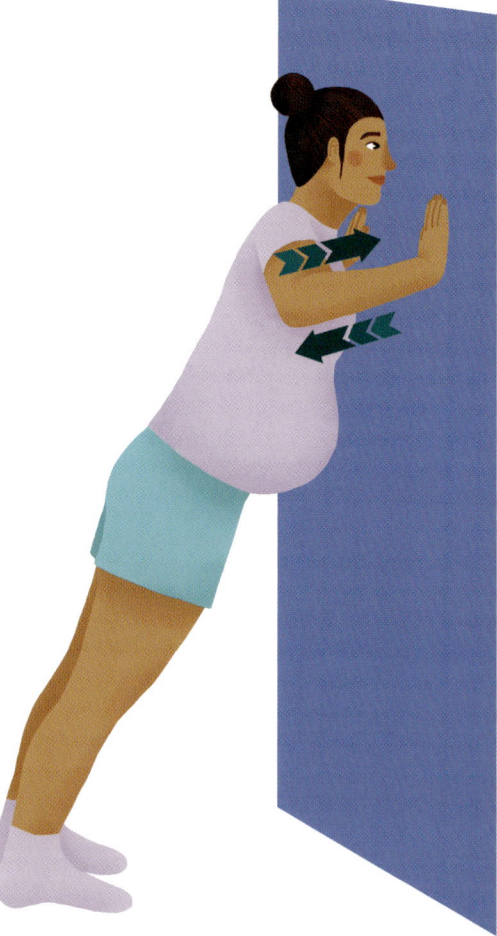

Acknowledgments

From Jessica Dorrington

To all the incredible moms I've had the privilege of walking alongside in their postpartum journeys, and to the future moms and practitioners who will continue to shape and transform this work—you each inspire me daily and are at the heart of its purpose.

A heartfelt thank you to my mentor, Taryn Hallam, PT, for keeping me informed and guiding our entire profession to higher levels of evidence-based care.

To my family, and especially my husband, thank you for your unwavering support as I pursued this passion during evenings and weekends.

To Shannon, my soul sister, whose endurance kept us going, your passion for sharing this knowledge fueled us, and your friendship blesses me every day.

To Avalon, who took our seven-year project and added the finesse needed to bring our vision to life.

And to the moms reading this book—you possess incredible strength and resilience, and it's an honor to accompany you on this monumental journey.

From Shannon Rowbury

This book is dedicated to all those who went before us. You paved the way that brought us here.

To my daughter, who inspired this book—you made me a mom, and through you, I discovered a new strength within myself. And to my son, whose birth gave me the motivation to make this book a reality.

To my mom—you were my first and most important example of what it means to be strong as a mother. And to my dad, whose quiet constancy and spirit of curiosity helped shape my worldview.

Special thanks to my husband, whose steadfast strength and love have made me braver.

To Jess, who stepped in as a guide when the road of being both an athlete and a mother felt especially rocky. Your wisdom forms the foundation of this book, and your joy has made this journey endlessly rewarding.

To our editor Avalon, for immediately understanding the need for this book. You poured yourself into this project, bringing it to life while simultaneously creating your beautiful daughter, whose spirit fills every page.

Published in association with the literary agency of Legacy, LLC, 501 N. Orlando Avenue, Suite #313-348, Winter Park, FL 32789.

References

The information in this book is based on current scientific research and clinical guidelines. Below is a comprehensive list of the academic and medical sources consulted in writing this book.

Agha, Riaz, Rei Ogawa, Giorgio Pietramaggiori, and Dennis P. Orgill. "A Review of the Role of Mechanical Forces in Cutaneous Wound Healing." *Journal of Surgical Research* 171, no. 2 (2011): 700–708.

Ahlqvist, Kerstin, Elisabeth Krefting Bjelland, Ronnie Pingel, et al. "Generalized Joint Hypermobility and the Risk of Pregnancy-Related Pelvic Girdle Pain: Is Body Mass Index of Importance?—A prospective Cohort Study." *Acta Obstetricia et Gynecologica Scandinavica* 102, no. 10 (2023): 1259–1268.

The American College of Obstetricians and Gynecologists, "Exercising During Pregnancy."

American Heart Association. "All About Heart Rate."

American Heart Association. "American Heart Association Recommendations for Physical Activity in Adults and Kids."

Artal, Raul, Victoria Fortunato, Ann Welton, et al. "A Comparison of Cardiopulmonary Adaptations to Exercise in Pregnancy at Sea Level and Altitude." *American Journal of Obstetrics & Gynecology* 172, no. 4 (1995): 1170–1180.

Ashton-Miller, James A., and John O. L. DeLancey. "Functional Anatomy of the Female Pelvic Floor." *Annals of the New York Academy of Sciences* 1101, no. 1 (2007): 266–296.

Barakat, Ruben, Evelia Franco, María Perales, Carmina López, and Michelle F. Mottola. "Exercise During Pregnancy Is Associated with a Shorter Duration of Labor. A Randomized Clinical Trial." *European Journal of Obstetrics & Gynecology and Reproductive Biology* 224 (2018): 33–40.

Barakat, Ruben, Mireia Pelaez, Carmina Lopez, Rocío Montejo, and Javier Coteron. "Exercise During Pregnancy Reduces the Rate of Cesarean and Instrumental Deliveries: Results of a Randomized Controlled Trial." *The Journal of Maternal-Fetal & Neonatal Medicine* 25, no. 11 (2012): 2372–2376.

Ben Ami, Nao, and Gali Dar. "What Is the Most Effective Verbal Instruction for Correctly Contracting the Pelvic Floor Muscles?" *Neurourology and Urodynamics* 37, no. 8 (2018): 2904–2910.

Benjamin, Deenika R., Helena C. Frawley, Nora Shields, Alexander T.M. van de Water, and Nicholas F. Taylor. "Relationship Between Diastasis of the Rectus Abdominis Muscle (DRAM) and Musculoskeletal Dysfunctions, Pain and Quality of Life: A Systematic Review." *Physiotherapy* 105, no. 1 (2019): 24–34.

Bixo, L., G. Sandblom, J. Österberg, O. Stackelberg, K. Bewö, and A. Olsson. "Association Between Inter-Recti Distance and Impaired Abdominal Core Function in Post-Partum Women with Diastasis Recti Abdominis." *Journal of Abdominal Wall Surgery* 1 (2022): 10909.

Blanco Gutiérrez, Verónica, Vanora A. Hundley, and Susan. Way. "The Experience of Women from Underrepresented Groups with Urinary Incontinence: A Systematic Review." *Journal of Transcultural Nursing* 34, no. 4 (2023): 288–300.

Blotta, Rosa Maria, Sirlei dos Santos Costa, Eduardo Neubarth Trindade, Luise Meurer, and Manoel Roberto Maciel-Trindade. "Collagen I and III in Women with Diastasis Recti." *Clinics* 73 (2018): e319.

Bø, Kari, and Jorunn Sundgot-Borgen. "Are Former Female Elite Athletes More Likely to Experience Urinary Incontinence Later in Life than Non-Athletes?" *Scandinavian Journal of Medicine & Science in Sports* 20, no. 1 (2010): 100–104.

Bø, Kari, Raul Artal, Ruben Barakat, et al. "Exercise and Pregnancy in Recreational and Elite Athletes: 2016 Evidence Summary from the IOC Expert Group Meeting, Lausanne. Part 2—the Effect of Exercise on the Fetus, Labour and Birth." *British Journal of Sports Medicine* 50, no. 21 (2016):1297–1305.

Bovbjerg Marit L., and Anna Maria Siega-Riz. "Exercise During Pregnancy and Cesarean Delivery: North Carolina PRAMS, 2004–2005." *Birth* 36, no. 3 (2009): 200–207.

Brennand, Erin, Eider Ruiz-Mirazo, Selphee Tang, and Shunaha Kim-Fine. "Urinary Leakage During Exercise: Problematic Activities, Adaptive Behaviors, and Interest in Treatment for Physically Active Canadian Women." *International Urogynecology Journal* 29, no. 4 (2018): 497–503.

Brooks, Kaylee C. L., Kevin Varette, Marie-Andrée Harvey, et al. "A Model Identifying Characteristics Predictive of Successful Pelvic Floor Muscle Training Outcomes Among Women with Stress Urinary Incontinence." *International Urogynecology Journal* 32, no. 3 (2021): 719–728.

Brunelli, Elena, Biancamaria Del Prete, Paolo Casadio, Gianluigi Pilu, and Aly Youssef. "The Dynamic Change of the Anteroposterior Diameter of the Levator Hiatus Under Valsalva Maneuver at Term and Labor Outcome." *Neurourology and Urodynamics* 39, no. 8 (2020): 2353–2360.

Burzynski, Bartlomiej, Tomasz Jurys, Michalina Knapik, et al. "Abdominal Complex Muscle in Women with Stress Urinary Incontinence—Prospective Case-Control Study." *Archives of Medical Science* 19, no. 4 (2021): 1016–1021.

Bužinskienė, Diana, Živilė Sabonytė-Balšaitienė, and Tomas Poškus. "Perianal Diseases in Pregnancy and After Childbirth: Frequency, Risk Factors, Impact on Women's Quality of Life and Treatment Methods." *Frontiers in Surgery* 9 (2022): 788823.

Bweir, Salameh, Muhammed Al-Jarrah, Abdul-Majeed Almalty, et al. "Resistance Exercise Training Lowers HbA1c More than Aerobic Training in Adults with Type 2 Diabetes." *Diabetology & Metabolic Syndrome* 1, no. 27 (2009).

Cabre, H. E., S.R. Moore, A. E. Smith-Ryan, and A. C. Hackney. "Relative Energy Deficiency in Sport (RED-S): Scientific, Clinical, and Practical Implications for the Female Athlete." *Deutsche Zeitschrift für Sportmedizin* 73, no. 7 (2022): 225–234.

Callahan, Elliott C., Won Lee, Pedram Aleshi, and Ronald B. George. "Modern Labor Epidural Analgesia: Implications for Labor Outcomes and Maternal-Fetal Health." *American Journal of Obstetrics and Gynecology* 228, no. 5 (2023): S1260—S1269.

Cammu, Hendrik, Michelle Van Nylen, Christophe Blockeel, Leon Kaufman, and Jean-Jacques Amy. "Who Will Benefit from Pelvic Floor Muscle Training for Stress Urinary Incontinence?" *American Journal of Obstetrics and Gynecology* 191, no. 4 (2004): 1152–1157.

Capel-Alcaraz, Ana María, Héctor García-López, Adelaida María Castro-Sánchez, Manuel Fernández-Sánchez, and Inmaculada Carmen Lara-Palomo. "The Efficacy of Strength Exercises for Reducing the Symptoms of Menopause: A Systematic Review." *Journal of Clinical Medicine* 12, no. 2 (2023): 548.

Cappelletti, Maurand, and Kim Wallen. "Increasing Women's Sexual Desire: The Comparative Effectiveness of Estrogens and Androgens." *Hormones and Behavior* 78 (2016): 178–93.

Carroll, Louise, Cliona O' Sullivan, Catherine Doody, Carla Perrotta, and Brona Fullen. "Pelvic Organ Prolapse: The Lived Experience." *PLOS One* 17, no. 11 (2022): e0276788.

Ceydeli, Adil, James Rucinski, and Leslie Wise. "Finding the Best Abdominal Closure: An Evidence-Based Review of the Literature." *Current Surgery* 62, no. 2 (2005): 220–225.

Charest, Jonathan, and Michael A. Grandner. "Sleep and Athletic Performance: Impacts on Physical Performance, Mental Performance, Injury Risk and Recovery, and Mental Health." *Sleep Medicine Clinics* 15, no. 1 (2020): 41–57.

Chen, Beibei, Xiumin Zhao, and Yan Hu. "Rehabilitations for Maternal Diastasis Recti Abdominis: An Update on Therapeutic Directions." *Heliyon* 9, no. 10 (2023): e20956.

Chidi-Ogbolu, Nkechinyere, and Keith Baar. "Effect of Estrogen on Musculoskeletal Performance and Injury Risk." *Frontiers in Physiology* 9 (2019): 1834.

Cho, Sung Tae, and Khae Hawn Kim. "Pelvic Floor Muscle Exercise and Training for Coping with Urinary Incontinence." *Journal of Exercise Rehabilitation* 17, no. 6 (2021): 379–387.

Chu, Christine M., Lily A. Arya, and Uduak U. Andy. "Impact of Urinary Incontinence on Female Sexual Health in Women During Midlife." *Women's Midlife Health* 1, no. 6 (2015).

Clapp, James F. "Influence of Endurance Exercise and Diet on Human Placental Development and Fetal Growth." *Placenta* 27, no. 6–7 (2006): 527–34.

Clapp, James F. "Morphometric and Neurodevelopmental Outcome at Age Five Years of the Offspring of Women Who Continued to Exercise Regularly Throughout Pregnancy." *The Journal of Pediatrics* 129, no. 6 (1996): 856–863.

Clapp, James F., and Catherine Cram. *Exercising Through Your Pregnancy.* 2nd ed. Addicus Books, 2012.

Clephane, Kirstin, and Tierney K. Lorenz. "Putative Mental, Physical, and Social Mechanisms of Hormonal Influences on Postpartum Sexuality." *Current Sexual Health Reports* 13, no. 4 (2021): 136–148.

Cleveland Clinic. "Round Ligament Pain."

Cody, June D., Madeleine Louisa Jacobs, Karen Richardson, Birgit Moehrer, and Andrew Hextall. "Oestrogen Therapy for Urinary Incontinence in Post-Menopausal Women." *The Cochrane Database of Systematic Reviews* 10 (2012): CD001405.

Correia, Rafael Ribeiro, Allice Santos Cruz Veras, William Rodrigues Tebar, Jéssica Costa Rufino, Victor Rogério Garcia Batista, and Giovana Rampazzo Teixeira. "Strength Training for Arterial Hypertension Treatment: A Systematic Review and Meta-Analysis of Randomized Clinical Trials." *Scientific Reports* 13, no. 201 (2023).

Côté, Emilie J.M., Madeleine Benton, Rachael Gardner, and Rachel Tribe. "Balancing Benefits and Risks of Exercise in Pregnancy: A Qualitative Analysis of Social Media Discussion." *BMJ Open Sport & Exercise Medicine* 10, no. 4 (2024): e002176.

Coyne, Sarah. M., Toni Liechty, Kevin M. Collier, Aubrey D. Sharp, Emilie J. Davis, and Savannah L. Kroff. "The Effect of Media on Body Image in Pregnant and Postpartum Women." *Health Communication* 33, no. 7 (2017): 793–799.

Damen, Léonie, H. Muzaffer Buyruk, Füsun Güler-Uysal, Frederik K. Lotgering, Chris J. Snijders, and Hendrik J. Stam. "The Prognostic Value of Asymmetric Laxity of the Sacroiliac Joints in Pregnancy-Related Pelvic Pain." *Spine* 27, no. 24 (2002): 2820–2824.

Damen, Léonie, H. Muzaffer Buyruk, Füsun Güler-Uysal, Frederik K. Lotgering, Chris J. Snijders, and Hendrik J. Stam. "Pelvic Pain During Pregnancy Is Associated with Asymmetric Laxity of the Sacroiliac Joints." *Acta Obstetricia Et Gynecologica Scandinavica* 80, no. 11 (2001): 1019–1024.

Davison, J. M. "Edema in Pregnancy." *Kidney International Supplement* 59 (1997): S90—S96.

Deering, Rita E., Meredith Cruz, Jonathon W. Senefeld, Tatyana Pashibin, Sarah Eickmeyer, and Sandra K. Hunter. "Impaired Trunk Flexor

Strength, Fatigability, and Steadiness in Postpartum Women." *Medicine & Science in Sports & Exercise* 50, no. 8 (2018): 1558–1569.

Dendini, Mohammad, Sara K. Aldossari, Hydar A. AlQassab, Othman O. Aldraihem, and Amwaj Almalki. "Retrospective Case-Control Study of Extended Birth Perineal Tears and Risk Factors." *Cureus* 16, no. 3 (2024): e57132.

Depledge, Jill, Peter McNair, and Richard Ellis. "Exercises, Tubigrip and Taping: Can They Reduce Rectus Abdominis Diastasis Measured Three Weeks Post-Partum?" *Musculoskeletal Science & Practice* 53 (2021): 102381.

Dietz, H. P., C. Shek, and B. Clarke. "Biometry of the Pubovisceral Muscle and Levator Hiatus by Three-Dimensional Pelvic Floor Ultrasound." *Ultrasound in Obstetrics & Gynecology* 25, no. 6 (2018): 580–585.

Dietz, Hans Peter. "Pelvic Floor Trauma in Childbirth." *The Australian & New Zealand Journal of Obstetrics & Gynaecology* 53, no. 3 (2013): 220–230.

DiFranco, Joyce T., and Marilyn Curl. "Healthy Birth Practice #5: Avoid Giving Birth on Your Back and Follow Your Body's Urge to Push." *The Journal of Perinatal Education* 23, no. 4 (2014): 207–210.

Dipietro, Loretta, Kelly R. Evenson, Bonny Bloodgood, et al. "Benefits of Physical Activity During Pregnancy and Postpartum: An Umbrella Review." *Medicine & Science in Sports & Exercise* 51, no. 6 (2019): 1292–1302.

Domenjoz, Iris, Bengt Kayser, and Michel Boulvain. "Effect of Physical Activity During Pregnancy on Mode of Delivery." *American Journal of Obstetrics and Gynecology* 211, no. 4 (2014): 401.e1-11.

Donnelly, Gráinne M., Isabel S. Moore, Emma Brockwell, Alan Rankin, and Rosalyn Cooke. "Reframing Return-to-Sport Postpartum: The 6 Rs Framework." *British Journal of Sports Medicine* 56, no. 5 (2022): 244–245.

Donnelly, G., E. Brockwell, and T. Goom. "Return to Running Postnatal— Guideline for Medical, Health and Fitness Professionals Managing This Population." *Physiotherapy* 107 (2020): e188—e189.

Drabiščáková, Paula, Júlia Hederlingová, Petra Oťapková, et al. "The Incidence and Risk Factors of Falls During Pregnancy." *Clinical and Experimental Obstetrics & Gynecology* 49, no. 5 (2022): 115.

Dufour, Sinéad P.T., Stéphanie Bernard, Beth Murray-Davis, and Nadine Graham. "Establishing Expert-Based Recommendations for the Conservative Management of Pregnancy-Related Diastasis Rectus Abdominis: A Delphi Consensus Study." *Journal of Women's & Pelvic Health Physical Therapy* 43, no. 2 (2019): 73–81.

Dumoulin, Chantale, Licia P. Cacciari, and E. J. C. Hay-Smith. "Pelvic Floor Muscle Training Versus No Treatment, or Inactive Control Treatments, for Urinary Incontinence in Women." *Cochrane Database of Systematic Reviews* 10 (2018): CD005654.

Emery, Jennifer, Nicole M. Book, and Joseph Novi. "The Association Between Post-Void Leakage and Coital Incontinence and Intrinsic Sphincter Deficiency Among Women with Urinary Incontinence." *Female Pelvic Medicine & Reconstructive Surgery* 16, no. 6 (2010): 349–352.

Evenson, Kelly R., Ruben Barakat, Wendy J. Brown, et al. "Guidelines for Physical Activity During Pregnancy: Comparisons from Around the World." *American Journal of Lifestyle Medicine* 8, no. 2 (2013): 102–121.

Evenson, Kelly R., Wendy J. Brown, Alison K. Brinson, Emily Budzynski-Seymour, and Melanie Hayman. "A Review of Public Health Guidelines for Postpartum Physical Activity and Sedentary Behavior from Around the World." *Journal of Sport and Health Science* 13, no. 4 (2024): 472–483.

Familiari, Alessandra, Caterina Neri, Elvira Passananti, et al. "Maternal Position During the Second Stage of Labor and Maternal-Neonatal Outcomes in Nulliparous Women: A Retrospective Cohort Study." *AJOG Global Reports* 3, no. 1 (2023): 100160.

Fede, Caterina, Carmelo Pirri, Chenglei Fan, et al. "Sensitivity of the Fasciae to Sex Hormone Levels: Modulation of Collagen-I, Collagen-III and Fibrillin Production." *PLOS One* 14, no. 9 (2019): e0223195.

Fitzgerald, Colleen M., Stacey Bennis, Marissa L. Marcotte, Megan B. Shannon, Sana Iqbal, and William H. Adams. "The Impact of a Sacroiliac Joint Belt on Function and Pain Using the Active Straight Leg Raise in Pregnancy-Related Pelvic Girdle Pain." *PM&R* 14, no. 1 (2021): 19–29.

Foster, Stefanie N., Theresa M Spitznagle, Lori J. Tuttle, et al. "Hip and Pelvic Floor Muscle Strength in Women with and without Urgency and Frequency Predominant Lower Urinary Tract Symptoms." *Journal of Women's Health Physical Therapy* 45, no. 3 (2021): 126–134.

Fradkin, Andrea J., Tsharni R. Zazryn, and James M. Smoliga. "Effects of Warming-Up on Physical Performance: A Systematic Review with Meta-Analysis." *Journal of Strength and Conditioning Research* 24, no. 1 (2010): 140–148.

Gilbert, Isabelle, Nathaly Gaudreault, and Isabelle Gaboury. "Exploring the Effects of Standardized Soft Tissue Mobilization on the Viscoelastic Properties, Pressure Pain Thresholds, and Tactile Pressure Thresholds of the Cesarean Section Scar." *Journal of Integrative and Complementary Medicine* 28, no. 4 (2022): 355–362.

Gluppe, Sandra B., Marie Ellström Engh, and Kari Bø. "Curl-Up Exercises Improve Abdominal Muscle Strength Without Worsening Inter-Recti Distance in Women with Diastasis Recti Abdominis Postpartum: A Randomised Controlled Trial." *Journal of Physiotherapy* 69, no. 3 (2023): 160–167.

Gluppe, Sandra B., Marie Ellström Engh, and Kari Bø. "Primiparous Women's Knowledge of Diastasis Recti Abdominis, Concerns About Abdominal Appearance, Treatments, and Perceived Abdominal Muscle Strength 6–8 Months Postpartum. A Cross Sectional Comparison Study." *BMC Women's Health* 22, no. 428 (2022).

Goldsmith, L.T., G. Weiss, and B.G. Steinetz. "Relaxin and Its Role in Pregnancy." *Endocrinology and*

Metabolism Clinics of North America 24, no. 1 (1995): 171–186.

González-Muñoz, Ana, Leo Pruimboom, and Santiago Navarro-Ledesma. "The Relationship Between the Elastic Properties and Pain Pressure Threshold in Cesarean Scar Tissue—An Observational Study." *Healthcare (Basel, Switzerland)* 12, no. 21 (2024): 2166.

Goodman, Janice H., and Lyda Tyer-Viola. "Detection, Treatment, and Referral of Perinatal Depression and Anxiety by Obstetrical Providers." *Journal of Women's Health* 19, no 3 (2010): 477–490.

Guinhouya, Benjamin C., Martine Duclos, Carina Enea, and Laurent Storme. "Beneficial Effects of Maternal Physical Activity during Pregnancy on Fetal, Newborn, and Child Health: Guidelines for Interventions during the Perinatal Period from the French National College of Midwives." *Journal of Midwifery & Women's Health* 67, no. S1 (2022): S149—S157.

Gunnarsson, Ulf, Birgit Stark, Ursula Dahlstrand, and Karin Strigård. "Correlation Between Abdominal Rectus Diastasis Width and Abdominal Muscle Strength." *Digestive Surgery* 32, no. 2 (2015): 112–116.

Haakstad, Lene A. H., and Kari Bø. "Exercise in Pregnant Women and Birth Weight: A Randomized Controlled Trial. BMC Pregnancy Childbirth." *BMC Pregnancy and Childbirth* 11, no. 66 (2011).

Hagen, Suzanne, Cathryn Glazener, Doreen McClurg, et al. "Pelvic Floor Muscle Training for Secondary Prevention of Pelvic Organ Prolapse (PREVPROL): A Multicentre Randomised Controlled Trial." *The Lancet* 389, no. 10067 (2017): 393–402.

Hagen, Suzanne, Diane Stark, Cathryn Glazener, et al. "Individualised Pelvic Floor Muscle Training in Women with Pelvic Organ Prolapse (POPPY): A Multicentre Randomised Controlled Trial." *The Lancet* 383, no. 9919 (2014): 796–806.

Handa, Victoria L., Joan L. Blomquist, Megan Carroll, Jennifer Roem, and Alvaro Muñoz. "Changes in the Genital Hiatus Preceding the Development of Pelvic Organ Prolapse." *American*

Journal of Epidemiology 188, no. 12 (2019): 2196–2201.

Harmanli, Oz. "POP-Q 2.0: Its Time Has Come!" *International Urogynecology Journal* 25, no. 4 (2014): 447–449.

Healthy Bones Australia. "Exercises for Osteoporosis."

Hinman, Sally K., Kristy B. Smith, David M. Quillen, and M. S. Smith. "Exercise in Pregnancy: A Clinical Review." *Sports Health* 7, no. 6 (2015): 527–531.

Hrvatin, Ivana, and Darja Rugelj. "Risk Factors for Accidental Falls During Pregnancy—a Systematic Literature Review." *The Journal of Maternal-Fetal & Neonatal Medicine* 35, no. 25 (2022): 7015–7024.

Huang, Kevin, and Joseph Ihm. "Sleep and Injury Risk." *Current Sports Medicine Reports* 20, no. 6 (2021): 286–290.

Iqbal, Jameel, and Mone Zaidi. "Understanding Estrogen Action During Menopause." *Endocrinology* 150, no. 8 (2009): 3443–3445.

Isenmann, Eduard, Dominik Kaluza, Tim Havers, et al. "Resistance Training Alters Body Composition in Middle-Aged Women Depending on Menopause—a 20-Week Control Trial." *BMC Women's Health* 23, no. 526 (2023.

Jackson, M. R., P. Gott, S. J. Lye, J. W. Ritchie, and J. F. Clapp 3rd. "The Effects of Maternal Aerobic Exercise on Human Placental Development: Placental Volumetric Composition and Surface Areas." *Placenta* 16, no. 2 (1995): 179–191.

Johns Hopkins Medicine. "Understanding Your Target Heart Rate."

Junginger, Baerbel, Hanna Vollhaber, and Kaven Baessler. "Submaximal Pelvic Floor Muscle Contractions: Similar Bladder-Neck Elevation, Longer Duration, Less Intra-Abdominal Pressure." *International Urogynecology Journal* 29, no. 11 (2018): 1681–1687.

Kalisiak, Brooke, and Theresa Spitznagle. "What Effect Does an Exercise Program for Healthy Pregnant Women Have on the Mother, Fetus, and Child?" *PM&R* 1, no. 3 (2009): 261–266.

Katz, Miriam. "Physical Activity During Pregnancy—Past and Present." *Developmental Period Medicine* 22, no. 1 (2018): 9–13.

Kaufmann, R.L., C. S. Reiner, U. A. Dietz, P. A. Clavien, R. Vonlanthen, and S. A. Käser. "Normal Width of the Linea Alba, Prevalence, and Risk Factors for Diastasis Recti Abdominis in Adults, a Cross-Sectional Study." *Hernia* 26, no. 2 (2022): 609–618.

Kawabata, Masashi, and Norihiro Shima. "Interaction of Breathing Pattern and Posture on Abdominal Muscle Activation and Intra-Abdominal Pressure in Healthy Individuals: A Comparative Cross-Sectional Study." *Scientific Reports* 13 (2023): 11338.

Kazma, Jamil M., John van den Anker, Karel Allegaert, André Dallmann, and Homa K. Ahmadzia. "Anatomical and Physiological Alterations of Pregnancy." *Journal of Pharmacokinetics and Pharmacodynamics* 47, no. 4 (2020): 271–285.

Keshwani, Nadia, Sunita Mathur, and Linda McLean. "The Impact of Exercise Therapy and Abdominal Binding in the Management of Diastasis Recti Abdominis in the Early Post-Partum Period: A Pilot Randomized Controlled Trial." *Physiotherapy Theory and Practice* 37, no. 9 (2021): 1018–1033.

Khunda, Azar, Ka Lai Shek, and Hans Peter Dietz. "Can Ballooning of the Levator Hiatus Be Determined Clinically?" *American Journal of Obstetrics and Gynecology* 206, no. 3 (2011): 246.e1–246.e2464.

Korevaar Tim I. M., Eric A. P. Steegers, Yolanda B. de Rijke, et al. "Reference Ranges and Determinants of Total hCG Levels During Pregnancy: The Generation R Study." *European Journal of Epidemiology* 30, no. 9 (2015): 1057–1066.

Krysiak, Robert, Agnieszka Drosdzol-Cop, Violetta Skrzypulec-Plinta, and Bogusław Okopien. "Sexual Function and Depressive Symptoms in Young Women with Elevated Macroprolactin Content: A Pilot Study." *Endocrine* 53, no. 1 (2016): 291–298.

Kuzawa, Christopher W., Lee T. Gettler, Yuan-yen Huang, and Thomas W. McDade. "Mothers Have Lower

Testosterone than Non-Mothers: Evidence from the Philippines." *Hormones and Behavior* 57, no. 4–5 (2010): 441–447.

La Leche League Canada "Sex, Hormones, and Breastfeeding."

Liaw, Lih-Jiun, Miao-Ju Hsu, Chien-Fen Liao, Mei-Fang Liu, and Ar-Tyan Hsu. "The Relationships Between Inter-Recti Distance Measured by Ultrasound Imaging and Abdominal Muscle Function in Postpartum Women: A 6-Month Follow-Up Study." *The Journal of Orthopaedic and Sports Physical Therapy* 41, no. 6 (2011): 435–443.

Liu, Laura X., and Zolt Arany. "Maternal Cardiac Metabolism in Pregnancy." *Cardiovascular Research* 101, no. 4 (2014): 545–553.

LoMauro, Antonella, and Andrea Aliverti. "Respiratory Physiology of Pregnancy: Physiology Masterclass." *Breathe (Sheffield)* 11, no. 4 (2015): 297–301.

MacArthur, C., D. Wilson, P. Herbison, et al. "Urinary Incontinence Persisting After Childbirth: Extent, Delivery History, and Effects in a 12-Year Longitudinal Cohort Study." *BJOG: An International Journal of Obstetrics & Gynaecology* 123, no. 6 (2016): 1022–1029.

Majchrzycki, Marian, Agnieszka Seremak-Mrozikiewicz, Aleksandra Kulczyk, and Joanna Lipiec. "Kinesiotherapy in Women After Gynecological Surgeries." *Menopause Review/ Przegląd Menopauzalny* 11, no. 6 (2012): 510-513.

Majchrzycki, Marian, Hubert Wolski, and Agnieszka Seremak-Mrozikiewicz. "Application of Osteopathic Manipulative Technique in the Treatment of Back Pain During Pregnancy." *Ginekologia Polska* 86, no. 3 (2015): 224–228.

Manchana, Tarinee, and Suvit Bunyavejchevin. "Impact on Quality of Life after Ring Pessary Use for Pelvic Organ Prolapse." *International Urogynecology Journal* 23, no. 7 (2012): 873–877.

Mazi, Baraa, Ouhoud Kaddour, and Ahmed Al-Badr. "Depression Symptoms in Women with Pelvic Floor Dysfunction: A Case-Control Study." *International Journal of Women's Health* 11 (2019): 143–148.

Mellett, Lauren Healey, and Gisele Bousquet. "Heart-Healthy Exercise." *Circulation* 127, no. 17 (2013).

Mens, J. M., A. Pool-Goudzwaard, and H. J. Stam. "Mobility of the Pelvic Joints in Pregnancy-Related Lumbopelvic Pain: A Systematic Review." *Obstetrical & Gynecological Survey* 64, no. 3 (2009): 200–208.

Meyer, R., A. Rottenstreich, M. Zamir, H. Ilan, E. Ram, M. Alcalay, and G. Levin. "Sonographic Fetal Head Circumference and the Risk of Obstetric Anal Sphincter Injury Following Vaginal Delivery." *International Urogynecology Journal* 31, no. 11 (2020): 2285–2290.

Miceli, A., M. Fernández-Sánchez, and J. L. Dueñas-Díez. "How Often Should Ring Pessaries Be Removed or Changed in Women with Advanced POP? A Prospective Observational Study." *International Urogynecology Journal* 32, no. 6 (2021): 1471–1478.

Momeni, Mazdak, Mohammad H. Rahbar, and Ertug Kovanci. "A Meta-Analysis of the Relationship between Endometrial Thickness and Outcome of In Vitro Fertilization Cycles." *Journal of Human Reproductive Sciences* 4, no. 3 (2011): 130–137.

Mota, Patrícia, Augusto Gil Pascoal, Ana Isabel Carita, and Kari Bø. "Normal Width of the Inter-Recti Distance in Pregnant and Postpartum Primiparous Women." *Musculoskeletal Science and Practice* 35 (2018): 34–37.

Mottola, Michelle F., Taniya S. Nagpal, Roberta Bgeginski, et al. "Is Supine Exercise Associated with Adverse Maternal and Fetal Outcomes? A Systematic Review." *British Journal of Sports Medicine* 53, no. 2 (2019): 82–89.

Mountjoy, M., J. Sundgot-Borgen, L. Burke, et al. "The IOC Relative Energy Deficiency in Sport Clinical Assessment Tool (RED-S CAT)." *British Journal of Sports Medicine* 49, no. 21 (2015): 1354.

Movalled, Kobra, Anis Sani, Leila Nikniaz, and Morteza Ghojazadeh. "The Impact of Sound Stimulations during Pregnancy on Fetal Learning: A Systematic Review." *BMC Pediatrics* 23, no. 183 (2023).

Muhleisen, Alicia. L., and Melissa M. Herbst-Kralovetz. "Menopause and the Vaginal Microbiome." *Maturitas* 91 (2016): 42–50.

Mukhtar, Nur Farihan, Beng Kwang Ng, Su Ee Phon, Mohamed Ismail Nor Azlin, Abdul Ghani Nur Azurah, and Pei Shan Lim. "Prevalence, Knowledge and Awareness of Pelvic Floor Disorder among Pregnant Women in a Tertiary Centre, Malaysia." *International Journal of Environmental Research and Public Health* 19, no. 14 (2022): 8314.

National Institute for Health and Care Excellence. "Urinary Incontinence and Pelvic Organ Prolapse in Women: Management."

National Institute of Health and Care Excellence. "Antenatal and Postnatal Mental Health: Clinical Management and Service Guidance."

National Institute of Mental Health. "Perinatal Depression."

Neels, Hedwig, Stefan De Wachter, Jean-Jacques Wyndaele, Michel Wyndaele, and Alexandra Vermandel. "Does Pelvic Floor Muscle Contraction Early After Delivery Cause Perineal Pain in Postpartum Women?" *European Journal of Obstetrics & Gynecology and Reproductive Biology* 208 (2017): 1–5.

Nemeth, Zoltan, Sándor Nagy, and Johannes Ott. "The Cube Pessary: An Underestimated Treatment Option for Pelvic Organ Prolapse? Subjective 1-Year Outcomes." *International Urogynecology Journal* 24, no. 10 (2013): 1695–1701.

Noel, Gordon L., Han K. Suh, Andrew G. Frantz. "Prolactin Release During Nursing and Breast Stimulation in Postpartum and Nonpostpartum Subjects." *The Journal of Clinical Endocrinology & Metabolism* 38, no. 3 (1974): 413–423.

Nygaard, Ingrid, Tammy Girts, Nancy H. Fultz, Kraig Kinchen, Gerhardt Pohl, and Barbara Sternfeld. "Is Urinary Incontinence a Barrier to Exercise in Women?" *Obstetrics & Gynecology* 106, no. 2 (2005): 307–314.

Oiye, Shadrack, Margaret Juma, Silvenus Konyole, and Fatuma Adan. "The Influence of Antenatal Oral Iron and Folic Acid Side Effects on Supplementation Duration in

Low-Resource Rural Kenya: A Cross-Sectional Study." *Journal of Pregnancy* 1 (2020): 9621831.

Orlando Health Women's Institute. "How Pregnancy Affects a Mother's Heart."

Pascual, Zoey N., and Michelle D. Langaker. "Physiology, Pregnancy."

Permatasari, Tria Astika Endah, and Amir Syafruddin. "The Relationship between Oxytocin Levels with Empathy and Breastfeeding Intention in Female Medical Students: A Cross-Sectional Study." *Annals of Medicine and Surgery (London)* 81 (2022): 104486.

Persinger, Rachel, Carl Foster, Mark Gibson, Dennis C. W. Fater, and John P. Porcari. "Consistency of the Talk Test for Exercise Prescription." *Medicine & Science in Sports & Exercise* 36 (2004): 1632–1636.

Poyatos-León, Raquel, Antonio García-Hermoso, Gema Sanabria-Martínez, Celia Álvarez-Bueno, Mairena Sánchez-López, and Vicente Martínez-Vizcaíno. "Effects of Exercise during Pregnancy on Mode of Delivery: A Meta-Analysis." *Acta Obstetricia et Gynecologica Scandinavica* 94, no. 10 (2015): 1039–1047.

Price, Bradley B., Saeid B. Amini, and Kaelyn Kappeler. "Exercise in Pregnancy: Effect on Fitness and Obstetric Outcomes—A Randomized Trial." *Medicine & Science in Sports & Exercise* 44, no. 12 (2012): 2263–2269.

Pritchard, J. A. "Changes in the Blood Volume during Pregnancy and Delivery." *Anesthesiology* 26 (1965): 393–399.

Qian, Xueya, Pin Li, Shaoqing Shi, Robert E. Garfield, and Huishu Liu. "Measurement of Uterine and Abdominal Muscle Electromyography in Pregnant Women for Estimation of Expulsive Activities during the 2nd Stage of Labor." *Gynecologic and Obstetric Investigation* 84, no. 6 (2019): 555–561.

Quiroz, Lieschen H., Alvaro Muñoz, Stuart H. Shippey, Robert E. Gutman, and Victoria L. Handa. "Vaginal Parity and Pelvic Organ Prolapse." *Journal of Reproductive Medicine* 55, no. 3–4 (2010): 93–98.

Rodríguez-Blanque, Raquel, Juan Carlos Sánchez-García, Antonio Manuel Sánchez-López, and María José

Aguilar-Cordero. "Physical Activity during Pregnancy and Its Influence on Delivery Time: A Randomized Clinical Trial." *PeerJ* 7 (2019): e6370.

Rute-Larrieta, Carmen, Gloria Mota-Cátedra, Juan Manuel Carmona-Torres, et al. "Physical Activity during Pregnancy and Risk of Gestational Diabetes Mellitus: A Meta-Review." *Life* 14, no. 6 (2024): 755.

Ryall, Stephanie, Heidi Ohrling, Trent Stellingwerff, Stephanie Black, Kristen Reilly, and Jane S. Thornton. "Contraception Choice for Female Endurance Athletes: What's Sport Got to Do With It? A Cross-Sectional Survey." *Sports Medicine* 54, no. 12 (2024): 3181–3197.

Sangsawang, Bussara, and Nucharee Sangsawang. "Stress Urinary Incontinence in Pregnant Women: A Review of Prevalence, Pathophysiology, and Treatment." *International Urogynecology Journal* 24, no. 6 (2013): 901–912.

Sartore, A., R. Pregazzi, P. Bortoli, E. Grimaldi, G. Ricci, and S. Guaschino. "The Urine Stream Interruption Test and Pelvic Muscle Function in the Puerperium." *International Journal of Gynaecology and Obstetrics* 78, no. 3 (2002): 235–239.

Schaffer, Joseph, and J. Andrew Fantl. "4 Urogenital Effects of the Menopause." *Baillière's Clinical Obstetrics and Gynaecology* 10, no. 3 (1996): 401–417.

Schlager, Angela, Kerstin Ahlqvist, Ronnie Pingel, Lena Nilsson-Wikmar, Christina B. Olsson, and Per Kristiansson. "Validity of the Self-Reported Five-Part Questionnaire as an Assessment of Generalized Joint Hypermobility in Early Pregnancy." *BMC Musculoskeletal Disorders* 21, no. 1 (2020): 514.

Schober, Justine M., and Donald Pfaff. "The Neurophysiology of Sexual Arousal." *Best Practice & Research Clinical Endocrinology & Metabolism* 21, no. 3 (2007): 445–461.

Sciore, Paul, Cyril B. Frank, and David A. Hart. "Identification of Sex Hormone Receptors in Human and Rabbit Ligaments of the Knee by Reverse Transcription-Polymerase Chain Reaction: Evidence That Receptors Are Present in Tissue from Both Male

and Female Subjects." *Journal of Orthopaedic Research* 16, no. 5 (1998): 604–610.

Segal, Neil A., Elizabeth R. Boyer, Patricia Teran-Yengle, Natalie A. Glass, Howard J. Hillstrom, and H. John Yack. "Pregnancy Leads to Lasting Changes in Foot Structure." *American Journal of Physical Medicine & Rehabilitation* 92, no. 3 (2013): 232–240.

Shakeel, Nilam, Kåre Rønn Richardsen, Egil W. Martinsen, Malin Eberhard-Gran, Kari Slinning, and Anne Karen Jenum. "Physical Activity in Pregnancy and Postpartum Depressive Symptoms in a Multiethnic Cohort." *Journal of Affective Disorders* 236 (2018): 93–100.

Shirazi, Talia N., Jennifer A. Bossio, David A. Puts, and Meredith L. Chivers. "Menstrual Cycle Phase Predicts Women's Hormonal Responses to Sexual Stimuli." *Hormones and Behavior* 103 (2018): 45–53.

Shorten, Allison, Jacki Donsante, and Brett Shorten. "Birth Position, Accoucheur, and Perineal Outcomes: Informing Women about Choices for Vaginal Birth." *Birth* 29, no. 1 (2002): 18–27.

Silbernagel, Karin Grävare, Roland Thomeé, Bengt I. Eriksson, and Jon Karlsson. "Continued Sports Activity, Using a Pain-Monitoring Model, During Rehabilitation in Patients with Achilles Tendinopathy: A Randomized Controlled Study." *The American Journal of Sports Medicine* 35, no. 6 (2007): 897–906.

Smith, Michelle D., Anne Russell, and Paul W. Hodges. "Disorders of Breathing and Continence Have a Stronger Association with Back Pain than Obesity and Physical Activity." *Australian Journal of Physiotherapy* 52, no. 1 (2006): 11–16.

Soma-Pillay, P., C. Nelson-Piercy, H. Tolppanen, and A. Mebazaa. "Physiological Changes in Pregnancy." *Cardiovascular Journal of Africa* 27, no. 2 (2016): 89–94.

Soultanakis, Helen N., Raul Artal, and Robert A. Wiswell. "Prolonged Exercise in Pregnancy: Glucose Homeostasis, Ventilatory and Cardiovascular Responses." *Seminars in Perinatology* 20, no. 4 (1996): 315–327.

Soultanakis-Aligianni, Helen N. "Thermoregulation During Exercise in Pregnancy." *Clinical Obstetrics and Gynecology* 46, no. 2 (2003): 442–455.

Spitznagle, Theresa M., Fah Che Leong, and Linda R. Van Dillen. "Prevalence of Diastasis Recti Abdominis in a Urogynecological Patient Population." *International Urogynecology Journal and Pelvic Floor Dysfunction* 18, no. 3 (2007): 321–328.

Stær-Jensen, Jette, Franziska Siafarikas, Gunvor Hilde, Jūratė Šaltytė Benth, Kari Bø, and Marie Ellström Engh. "Postpartum Recovery of Levator Hiatus and Bladder Neck Mobility in Relation to Pregnancy." *Obstetrics & Gynecology* 125, no. 3 (2015): 531–539.

Stanford Medicine. "Edinburgh Postnatal Depression Scale (EPDS)."

Starzec-Proserpio, Małgorzata, Montserrat Rejano-Campo, Agata Szymańska, Jacek Szymański, and Barbara Baranowska. "The Association Between Postpartum Pelvic Girdle Pain and Pelvic Floor Muscle Function, Diastasis Recti and Psychological Factors: A Matched Case-Control Study." *International Journal of Environmental Research and Public Health* 19, no. 10 (2022): 6236.

Sutherland, Lauren Q. C. "The Right of Patients to Make Autonomous Choices: *Montgomery V Lanarkshire Health Board*: A Landmark Decision on Information Disclosure to Patients in the UK." *International Urogynecology Journal* 32, no. 7 (2021): 2005–2010.

The American College of Obstetricians and Gynecologists. "Exercise During Pregnancy: Frequently Asked Questions."

The American College of Obstetricians and Gynecologists. "How Much Weight Should I Gain During Pregnancy?"

Theodorsen, Nina-Margrethe, Kari Bø, Kjartan Vibe Fersum, Inger Haukenes, and Rolf Moe-Nilssen. "Pregnant Women May Exercise Both Abdominal and Pelvic Floor Muscles During Pregnancy Without Increasing the Diastasis Recti Abdominis: A Randomised Trial." *Journal of Physiotherapy* 70, no. 2 (2024): 142–148.

Ting, Alison Y., Audrey D. Blacklock, and Peter G. Smith. "Estrogen Regulates Vaginal Sensory and Autonomic Nerve Density in the Rat." *Biology of Reproduction* 71, no. 4 (2004): 1397–1404.

Tuominen, Reetta, Tiina Jahkola, Jani Mikkonen, Hannu Luomajoki, Jari Arokoski, and Jaana Vironen. "Low Back Pain and Motor Control Dysfunction After Pregnancy: The Possible Role of Rectus Diastasis." *International Journal of Abdominal Wall and Hernia Surgery* 6, no. 1 (2023): 30–36.

U.S. Centers for Disease Control and Prevention. "Breastfeeding Benefits Both Baby and Mom."

Uvnäs Moberg, Kerstin, Anette Ekström-Bergström, Sarah Buckley, et al. "Maternal Plasma Levels of Oxytocin During Breastfeeding—A Systematic Review." *PLOS One* 15, no. 8 (2020): e0235806.

Van Poppel, Mireille N. M., Annika Kruse, and Anthony M. Carter. "Maternal Physical Activity in Healthy Pregnancy: Effect on Fetal Oxygen Supply." *Acta Physiologica* 240, no. 11 (2024): e14229.

Vargas-Terrones, Marina, Ruben Barakat, Belen Santacruz, Irene Fernandez-Buhigas, and Michelle F. Mottola. "Physical Exercise Programme During Pregnancy Decreases Perinatal Depression Risk: A Randomised Controlled Trial." *British Journal of Sports Medicine* 53, no. 6 (2019): 348–353.

Vargas-Terrones, Marina, Taniya S. Nagpal, and Ruben Barakat. "Impact of Exercise During Pregnancy on Gestational Weight Gain and Birth Weight: An Overview." *Brazilian Journal of Physical Therapy* 23, no. 2 (2019): 164–169.

Vesting, Sabine, Annelie Gutke, and Monika Fagevik Olsén. "Can Clinical Postpartum Muscle Assessment Help Predict the Severity of Postpartum Pelvic Girdle Pain? A Prospective Cohort Study." *Physical Therapy* 103, no. 1 (2022): pzac152.

Viktrup, L., and G. Lose. "The risk of stress incontinence 5 years after first delivery." *American Journal of Obstetrics and Gynecology* 185, no. 1 (2001): 82–87.

Watkins, Virginia Y., Carly M. O'Donnell, Marta Perez, et al. "The Impact of Physical Activity During Pregnancy on Labor and Delivery." *American Journal of Obstetrics and Gynecology* 225, no. 4 (2021): 437.e1–437.e8.

Woodley, Sarah J., Philippa Lawrenson, Rachel Boyle, et al. "Pelvic Floor Muscle Training for Preventing and Treating Urinary and Faecal Incontinence in Antenatal and Postnatal Women." *Cochrane Database of Systematic Reviews* 5 (2020): CD007471.

World Health Organization. "Breastfeeding."

Yee, Lynn M., Anjali J. Kaimal, Sanae Nakagawa, Kathryn Houston, and Miriam Kuppermann. "Predictors of Postpartum Sexual Activity and Function in a Diverse Population of Women." *Journal of Midwifery & Women's Health* 58, no. 6 (2013): 654–61.

Zhang, Chenchen, Lixiang Li, Biying Jin, et al. "The Effects of Delivery Mode on the Gut Microbiota and Health: State of Art." *Frontiers in Microbiology* 12 (2021): 724449.

Zhang, Hongyu, Shurong Huang, Xiaolan Guo, et al. Comparing Maternal and Neonatal Outcomes Between Hands-and-Knees Delivery Position and Supine Position." *International Journal of Nursing Sciences* 3, no. 2 (2016): 178–184.

Zorzano, Antonio, Manuel Palacín, and X. Testar. "Insulin Resistance in Pregnancy." In *Perinatal Biochemistry*. CRC Press, 1992.

Index

About the Authors

Shannon Rowbury is one of the most accomplished middle-distance runners in U.S. history: a three-time Olympian and Olympic bronze medalist who set American, Area, and World records during her career. Ranked among the world's top ten for a decade, she brings elite athletic insight and deep understanding of performance across all life stages.

A trailblazer for athlete mothers, Shannon created the first-ever US Sports National Governing Body Maternity Policy in 2018 for USA Track & Field, revolutionizing support for pregnant and postpartum athletes. Beyond the track, she is a respected speaker, sports broadcaster, and creator of Medalist Mindset, a leadership framework that translates Olympic performance tools into strategies for personal and professional growth. She earned an Emmy for her work with NBC as a Distance Analyst for the 2024 Olympic coverage.

A Duke University graduate with both undergraduate and master's degrees (with honors), Shannon also holds executive education certificates from Harvard Business School, the Tuck School of Business at Dartmouth, and IMD. As a Sports Envoy for the US Department of State, she has led international workshops using sport to build connection and leadership across cultures. As an athlete, mother, and advocate for women's health, Shannon brings an authoritative voice to the intersection of sport, pregnancy, and postpartum wellness.

Jessica Dorrington, PT, MPT, OCS, CMPT, PRPC, PCES is a highly regarded Physical Therapist specializing in the intersection of pelvic floor health, orthopedics, athletics, and sports performance. Based in Portland, Oregon, she has empowered countless women since 2002, particularly during pregnancy and postpartum, while also consulting with professional athletes and addressing the unique challenges in pelvic health during these critical phases, from amateur to elite levels.

As a shareholder and director with Therapeutic Associates, Inc., Jessica has cultivated one of the largest pelvic health practices in the country. Board certified as an Orthopedic Specialist and certified as a Manual Physical Therapist, Pelvic Floor Rehabilitation Practitioner, Postpartum Corrective Exercise Specialist, and formerly a Certified Strength and Conditioning Specialist, she brings comprehensive expertise to maternal health.

Jessica is committed to mentoring future pelvic health practitioners and lecturing within the medical community to expand access and resources for maternal pelvic health. An avid runner herself, she understands the importance of exercise for mothers and applies her Strong as a Mother approach to her own postpartum athletic pursuits. She has set personal records in the 5K, 10K, Half Marathon, and Marathon (2:56:02) postpartum, qualifying for the Boston Marathon and placing 10th at the Age Group World Championships Marathon Race. Her mission is equipping women with tools to be proactive in their health and excel in both athletic pursuits and everyday life.

Copyright © 2026 by Shannon Rowbury and Jessica Dorrington
Illustrations copyright © 2026 by Michaela Hobson

Printed in China

SASQUATCH BOOKS with colophon is a registered trademark
of Blue Star Press, LLC.

30 29 28 27 26   9 8 7 6 5 4 3 2 1

Editor: Avalon Radys
Production editor: Peggy Gannon
Designer: Anna Goldstein

Library of Congress Cataloging-in-Publication Data is available.

ISBN: 978-1-63217-581-6

Sasquatch Books
1325 Fourth Avenue, Suite 1025
Seattle, WA 98101

SasquatchBooks.com

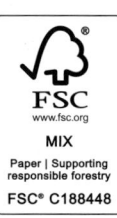

*The information contained in this book is intended for general
informational purposes only and does not constitute medical
advice. It is not a substitute for professional medical evaluation,
diagnosis, or treatment. Always seek the advice of your physician
or other qualified health provider with any questions you may
have regarding a medical condition or treatment, particularly
concerning exercise during pregnancy. The author and publisher
assume no responsibility for any adverse effects or consequences
resulting from the use of the information contained in this book.*

FSC
www.fsc.org
MIX
Paper | Supporting
responsible forestry
FSC® C188448